D0209586

Obsessive-Compulsive Disorder Casebook

Revised Edition

NATIONAL UNIVERSITY
LIBRARY   SAN DIEGO

Obsessive-Compulsive Disorder Casebook

Revised Edition

John H. Greist, M.D.
Distinguished Senior Scientist
Dean Foundation for Health, Research and Education;
Clinical Professor of Psychiatry
University of Wisconsin Medical School
Madison, Wisconsin

James W. Jefferson, M.D.
Distinguished Senior Scientist
Dean Foundation for Health, Research and Education;
Clinical Professor of Psychiatry
University of Wisconsin Medical School
Madison, Wisconsin

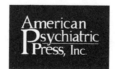

American
Psychiatric
Press, Inc.

Washington, DC
London, England

Note: The authors have worked to ensure that all information in this book concerning drug dosages, schedules, and routes of administration is accurate as of the time of publication and consistent with standards set by the U.S. Food and Drug Administration and the general medical community. As medical research and practice advance, however, therapeutic standards may change. For this reason and because human and mechanical errors sometimes occur, we recommend that readers follow the advice of a physician who is directly involved in their care or the care of a member of their family.

Books published by the American Psychiatric Press, Inc., represent the views and opinions of the individual authors and do not necessarily represent the policies and opinions of the Press or the American Psychiatric Association.

Copyright © 1995 American Psychiatric Press, Inc.
ALL RIGHTS RESERVED
Manufactured in the United States of America on acid-free paper
98 97 96 95   4 3 2 1
Second Edition

American Psychiatric Press, Inc.
1400 K Street, N.W., Washington, DC   20005

This book was sponsored by the University of Wisconsin Medical School, Continuing Medical Education, and made possible by an educational grant from Ciba-Geigy.

Library of Congress Cataloging-in-Publication Data
Obsessive-compulsive disorder casebook / by John H. Greist,
    James W. Jefferson. — 2nd Edition
        p.   cm.
    Includes bibliographical references and index.
    ISBN 0-88048-729-1 (alk. paper)
    1. Obsessive-compulsive disorder—Diagnosis—Case studies.
I. Greist, John H. II. Jefferson, James W.
    [DNLM: 1. Obsessive-Compulsive Disorder—diagnosis—case studies.
WM 176 0143 1995]
RC533.0265 1995
616.85′227—dc20
DNLM/DLC
for Library of Congress   94-41299
                                                                          CIP
British Library Cataloguing in Publication Data
A CIP record is available from the British Library.

CONTENTS

CLINICIAN CONTRIBUTORS

The authors wish to express appreciation to all those clinicians who contributed case histories to this book. Specifically, we thank the following individuals:

Jambur Ananth, M.D.
James M. Bailey, M.D., P.A.
Albert M. Bromberg, M.D.
Paul A. Buongiorno, M.D.
Jerome Char, M.D.
Reuven Dar, Ph.D.
Krishna Das Gupta, M.D.
Roberto A. Dominguez, M.D.
Robert L. Fischer, M.D., P.A.
Mark S. Friedlander, M.D.
Wayne K. Goodman, M.D.
Da-Shih Hu, M.D.
Hugh F. Johnston, M.D.
Han Soo Lee, M.D.
John S. March, M.D., M.P.H.
Habib Nathan, M.D.
Alan H. Peck, M.D., P.A.
Steven A. Rasmussen, M.D.
Scott Rauch, M.D.
William H. Young, Jr., M.D.
John M. Zajecka, M.D.

The *Obsessive-Compulsive Disorder Casebook* was first distributed in installments in 1991 and 1992 by Ciba-Geigy to physicians and psychologists. The casebook was well received, and we are pleased that the American Psychiatric Press has decided to publish the cases in book form and that the American Medical Association is continuing to offer CME credit through the University of Wisconsin to readers who take the tests at the end of each chapter.

We would like to express our deep appreciation to Ciba-Geigy for providing educational grants to cover the expense of developing, publishing, and disseminating the original casebook and for consenting to the publication of this new version. Ciba-Geigy's willingness to underwrite the cost of a large educational program in which the focus is on diagnosis, not pharmacotherapy, and in which there is no mention of their products or those of any other pharmaceutical manufacturer is laudable. Specifically, we would like to thank those at Ciba-Geigy who helped in the development and execution of the original casebook, namely, Joseph DeVeaugh-Geiss, M.D.; Rama Seshamani, M.D.; Carroll W. (Bo) Allen; Bruce Rowan; Carlos O. Stalgis; and Robert E. Killen.

Our thanks to Ann Bailey at the University of Wisconsin, who handled all the details associated with CME accreditation for the original program and for this book. We also wish to thank Lynn Tobias at the Dean Foundation for typing portions of the manuscript. Cathy Somer converted the separate sections into a coherent whole and created indices and new front matter for this edition. Finally, we wish to thank the many psychiatrists and psychologists from across the country who contributed the fascinating and varied case histories that constitute this casebook. Their interest and enthusiastic assistance were essential to the project.

We hope that those of you who are reading these cases for the first time will find them helpful in sharpening your understanding of obsessive-compulsive disorder and its comorbid and related conditions. The recognition and treatment of this fascinating disorder are gratifying to both physicians and patients.

John H. Greist, M.D.
James W. Jefferson, M.D.

Obsessive-compulsive disorder (OCD) has intrigued so many of us because it is about people, the tragic waste of their lives, and the long history of misunderstanding of this illness. Studying OCD has been one of the finest scientific adventures of my career, sending me into work with a variety of conditions and research strategies, and opening up surprising, new medical and neurological avenues for investigation. But the driving force behind all this work has been the patients with their fascinating stories and their enthusiasm and relief upon recognition of their plight.

This book is the result of a popular case series initially distributed to physicians and psychologists as part of an educational effort to increase diagnosis and treatment of OCD. There can be no better way to do it! My own fascination with the disorder derives from the lucidity of patients with OCD, the particular flavor of their descriptions of their symptoms, their bewilderment at their own rituals and repetitive thoughts, and their varied explanations for these symptoms.

This casebook goes into virtually all the manifestations of OCD, including its various symptoms such as doubting and hoarding, as well as comorbidity and differential diagnosis. Subtle points, such as the puzzling but inconsistent relationship between OCD symptoms and the menstrual cycle, and the coexistence of OCD and trichotillomania, are all here. The authors' impressive cumulative experience and that of the many colleagues who contributed cases to this book are evident. Anyone reading through this casebook will be aware of the complexity of the process of differentiating OCD from, for example, depression, phobia, eating disorders, or psychosis. The relationship of OCD to tic disorders and self-injurious behavior is particularly well illustrated (see Case Presentation 3).

None of my remarks convey the clarity and good judgment used in presenting these cases. They are just right in length and complexity.

The authors have really outdone themselves wih the continuing medical education (CME) questions provided at the end of each chapter. These questions are much more thought provoking than the usual CME questions hurriedly thrown together for this sort of exercise.

So welcome to another fascinating and instructive cast of characters in the OCD saga. This adventure will never end.

Judith L. Rapoport, M.D.

Comorbidity and
Obsessive-Compulsive Disorder

There is increasing interest and activity in psychiatric nosology, and new editions of the *Diagnostic and Statistical Manual of Mental Disorders* (DSM) arrived ever more rapidly through DSM-III but now seem settled into a 7-year cycle: DSM-I, 1952; DSM-II, 1968; DSM-III, 1980; DSM-III-R, 1987; DSM-IV, 1994.

Although we applaud DSM-III,[1] DSM-III-R,[2] and DSM-IV[3] for the greater interrater reliability they have brought to psychiatric diagnosis, we recognize that crisp diagnostic dichotomies correspond only crudely with clinical circumstances. From DSM-III to DSM-III-R, many hierarchies that prohibited comorbidity were eliminated. Furthermore, both DSM-III and DSM-III-R state that "there is no assumption that each mental disorder is a discrete entity with sharp boundaries (discontinuity) between it and other mental disorders, or between it and no mental disorder."[4] In DSM-IV, this

[1] American Psychiatric Association: *Diagnostic and Statistical Manual of Mental Disorders*, 3rd Edition. Washington, D.C., American Psychiatric Association, 1980.

[2] American Psychiatric Association: *Diagnostic and Statistical Manual of Mental Disorders*, 3rd Edition, Revised. Washington, D.C., American Psychiatric Association, 1987.

[3] American Psychiatric Association: *Diagnostic and Statistical Manual of Mental Disorders*, 4th Edition. Washington, D.C., American Psychiatric Association, 1994.

[4] American Psychiatric Association: *Diagnostic and Statistical Manual of Mental Disorders*, 3rd Edition, Revised. Washington, D.C., American Psychiatric Association, 1987, p. xxii.

concept is continued: "There is no assumption that each category of mental disorder is a completely discrete entity with absolute boundaries dividing it from other mental disorders or from no mental disorder."[5]

The clinical world is overlapping and continuous rather than discrete and categorical. Our quest for greater diagnostic homogeneity should not interfere with clinical realities of comorbidity and disorder spectra or with our comfort and confidence in recognizing, acknowledging, and treating them.

Regarding obsessive-compulsive disorder (OCD), in DSM-III-R, "some activities, such as eating (e.g., eating disorders), sexual behavior (e.g., paraphilias), gambling (e.g., pathological gambling), or drinking (e.g., alcohol dependence or abuse)" were excluded from being "true compulsions because the person derives pleasure from the particular activity, and may wish to resist it only because of its secondary deleterious consequences."[6] There was recognition that behaviors associated with these disorders "when engaged in excessively may be referred to as 'compulsive.'" Also excluded were ruminations occurring in the context of depressive disorders even though they have an obvious "obsessional" quality. When strictly observed, these exclusion criteria yield more homogeneous populations with presumably "pure" OCD.

Imposition of rigid boundaries between disorders may obscure common pathophysiological processes underlying them. Thus, dysmorphophobia, depersonalization, somatization, hypochondriasis, posttraumatic stress disorder, and eating disorders share with OCD an obsessional preoccupation with harm. Patients have an excessive worry about risks that most persons view as small or unavoidable. Persons with OCD often feel compelled to perform ritualistic behaviors to lessen their worry. Trichotillomania and onychophagia (i.e., nail biting) are characterized by their persistence across years and

[5] American Psychiatric Association: *Diagnostic and Statistical Manual of Mental Disorders*, 4th Edition. Washington, D.C., American Psychiatric Association, 1994, p. xxii.

[6] American Psychiatric Association: *Diagnostic and Statistical Manual of Mental Disorders*, 3rd Edition, Revised. Washington, D.C., American Psychiatric Association, 1987, p. 246.

by being "habits" done in a somewhat "absent-minded" manner.

As recognized in DSM-III-R, paraphilias and some impulse control disorders (kleptomania, pyromania, and pathological gambling—trichotillomania is also classified here) often include a "compulsive" quality. Persons with these disorders may also complain of intrusive obsessional thinking about their compulsive behaviors.

DSM-IV reflects recent recognition of the common comorbidity of obsessive-compulsive spectrum disorders. The DSM-IV criteria require only that

> if another Axis I disorder is present, the content of the obsessions or compulsions is not restricted to it (e.g., preoccupation with food in the presence of an Eating Disorder; hair pulling in the presence of Trichotillomania; concern with appearance in the presence of Body Dysmorphic Disorder; preoccupation with drugs in the presence of Substance Use Disorder; preoccupation with having a serious illness in the presence of Hypochondriasis; preoccupation with sexual urges or fantasies in the presence of a Paraphilia; or guilty ruminations in the presence of Major Depressive Disorder).[7]

Case Selection

The cases in this book represent some of the intuitively self-evident comorbidity and spectrum overlaps in diagnosis in order to make them more manifest. Our goal is to increase our comfort with what we already know to give us confidence to extend these concepts, when appropriate, to our patients' problems.

Cases were selected to reflect a wide range of OCD presentations, comorbidity, and obsessive-compulsive spectrum disorders that often create diagnostic confusion. The selected cases have been

[7]American Psychiatric Association: *Diagnostic and Statistical Manual of Mental Disorders*, 4th Edition. Washington, D.C., American Psychiatric Association, 1994, p. 423.

modified to protect confidentiality. We have exercised our best judgment in discussing these cases but recognize that there is room for disagreement with our conclusions.

Diagnoses and Editing

The diagnoses from the first edition of this casebook have been revised to make them consistent with those in DSM-IV. Axis I diagnoses are presented in order of importance, and diagnoses on other axes, where appropriate, are presented in numerical sequence. Other emendations have also been made where appropriate.

Indexes

In addition to a subject index, two other indexes are provided, one consisting of the case history titles and numbers, and the other, of all the diagnoses that appear in the 60 cases. The latter index will be especially useful for readers who wish to study various presentations of a certain diagnosis.

Educational Objectives

Through participation in this program, you will be better able

1. To discriminate between OCD and other conditions with symptoms overlapping those of OCD.
2. To assess the relative diagnostic importance (e.g., primary or secondary diagnosis) of various comorbid psychiatric disorders in a patient-specific context.

3. To apply DSM-IV criteria to cases involving OCD.
4. To discover OCD-like behavior in patients who present with other problems and to determine whether OCD is a valid diagnosis in those cases.

Continuing Medical Education Credit

Readers of this book who wish to earn American Medical Association (AMA) Category I credit or Continuing Medical Education (CME) credit may do so by answering the CME questions provided at the end of each chapter, noting their answers on the corresponding answer sheets in the accompanying booklet, and mailing the answer sheets to the University of Wisconsin for processing, along with a check covering the application fee, as explained in the accompanying booklet. Three hours of AMA Category I credit or CME hours or units will be awarded for the satisfactory completion of each set of 12 questions for a single chapter. Readers need not apply for all 30 credits unless they wish, in which case they need to answer all 120 questions.

ACCME

The University of Wisconsin is accredited by the Accreditation Council for Continuing Medical Education to sponsor CME for physicians.

AMA/PRA

The University of Wisconsin designates this CME activity for up to 30 credit hours in Category I of the Physician's Recognition Award of the American Medical Association.

Continuing Education Units

This program is accredited by the University of Wisconsin, Continuing Medical Education, for 3.0 CEUs (30 hours).

Please note: You may not apply for CME credit for any portion of the *Obsessive-Compulsive Disorder Casebook* for which you already earned CME credit under the original program.

Case Presentation 1
How Do I Know It Is Normal?

When Robert is referred for an evaluation, he is in his mid-30s and has a bright career ahead. He is a practicing radiologist, a few years out of a very competitive medical school from which he had graduated in the top third of his class. Robert was referred by an experienced general psychiatrist principally because of his compulsive symptoms, which are increasingly interfering with Robert's practice and social life.

Robert's compulsions emerged almost 2 years before the initial consultation, just after the death of a close relative. This relative had informally consulted with him a few months before her death. She had complained of persistent gastrointestinal distress and abdominal discomfort. To this description Robert added, "It was unusual for her to voice any complaints. She was relatively young and had always been in good health. . . . I took her symptoms very seriously." Robert examined her and ordered some laboratory and X-ray procedures at his office. When all test results proved negative, he reassured his relative and prescribed symptomatic treatment. Her symptoms continued, and within a few weeks she began to lose weight, looked as if she had aged several years, and was unable to keep food down. A reevaluation revealed an inoperable malignancy. The course of her illness was rapid; within a month she was dead.

After her death Robert reviewed her original X-ray films. He carefully noted the position of her gastrointestinal organs and said to himself, "Perhaps if I had looked at this area more meticulously . . . indeed, there is a suggestion of an anatomical distortion . . . she

1

could be alive today." As this "doubt" emerged, Robert began to doubt all his judgments.

During the interview Robert monotonously describes how painful it is now to read a normal chest X-ray film: "I have interpreted thousands of X-ray films before . . . now I can't finish one. I will read the film the usual way and recognize that it is normal. Then I will ask myself how I know that it is normal . . . Does the mediastinum seem normal? . . . Are the costophrenic angles as sharp as they should be? . . . Are there any hairline fractures? . . . Is that the right nipple or a soft tissue mass? I can't read *one* X-ray film. My partners know there is something wrong. I ask them to let me do all the other procedures."

Robert's symptoms are affecting his family and marital life as well. During the past few months his depression has intensified. It is now a chore to escort his wife to a restaurant or to a gathering with his colleagues. Robert and his wife had enjoyed a strong and positive relationship, but now they are drifting apart. His wife knows about his worries, and, like everyone in his family, she thinks that his concerns are nonsense and that the death was inevitable. Yet, Robert feels severe guilt.

As the interview progresses, it is difficult to be certain about Robert's diagnosis. Over the last few months, intensive psychotherapy and pharmacotherapy focusing principally on the depression have been of little help. His compulsive symptoms clearly preceded his dysphoric mood, although currently his depressive symptoms are just as severe.

DSM-IV Diagnoses

Axis I: 300.3   Obsessive-Compulsive Disorder

296.2x   Major Depressive Disorder, Single Episode

Discussion

One of the most common challenges for the clinician is differentiating patients with primary depression from those with obsessive-compulsive disorder (OCD). Major depression and OCD commonly coexist. Although the depression is often secondary to the OCD, as many as 30% of patients with OCD may also have a primary depressive disorder. Moreover, the symptoms of depressed patients may be misleading. Depressed melancholic patients often report inappropriate guilty ruminations, depersonalization, and, occasionally, delusional symptoms that may be mistaken for obsessions. These patients can also present with obsessional and, more frequently, compulsive symptoms. Similarly, because of the chronicity of their symptoms and the resulting social and vocational impairment and demoralization, patients with OCD often present with concomitant depressive symptoms.

There are several atypical features about the onset and duration of Robert's symptoms for a diagnosis of OCD. It is unusual for patients with OCD to relate the emergence of their symptoms to a specific event. In addition, the total duration of Robert's symptoms was relatively short. Most patients with OCD present for treatment in their late 20s to early 40s and date the onset of their symptoms to adolescence or early adulthood. In spite of these atypical features, the emergence of Robert's compulsive symptoms before his dysphoric mood, together with the nature of his obsessive doubting and resultant checking behavior, justifies a primary diagnosis of OCD, with depression secondary to the OCD.

Case Presentation 2
The Wastebasket Apartment

Kim, a 31-year-old unmarried woman, was referred to the clinic by a female acquaintance who had become concerned about the accumulation of things in Kim's apartment. Kim herself says that she has kept some of the objects that clutter her apartment for sentimental reasons. She is vague, however, in explaining how her apartment has become full of tissues, junk mail, and old newspapers, which she finds difficult to discard. She comments that she seems to use her apartment as "something between a wastebasket and a suitcase." She reports that the current situation is better than it was before her recent move to her new apartment. When preparing for the move, she was able to discard about eight garbage bags full of objects she had accumulated.

A more prominent concern for Kim is her difficulty coping with feelings of anxiety, which she experiences mainly in social situations in which she worries that her anxiety will be noticed by others. As a result, she avoids situations in which she might be a focus of attention. She feels anxious in enclosed places and crowded buses. She is especially uncomfortable standing in line at the grocery store, because she dreads the feeling that others are impatiently waiting for her to complete her transaction. She experiences great difficulty in making decisions, and anything outside her usual routine, such as taking the bus to the clinic today, seems overwhelmingly complex.

Kim reports a long history of social isolation and difficulties in interpersonal relationships. She has never had close friends or intimate relationships, and she has always felt like an outsider at social gatherings. For the past 7 years she has worked at an insurance company, doing filing in relative social isolation. She has always been extremely sensitive to real or imagined rejection. When her brother did not follow up on his promise to meet with her on her birthday, the hurt and the sense of disappointment she felt stayed with her for an entire year. In the past, such experiences triggered in Kim periods of despair and thoughts of suicide, but she has never attempted to hurt herself. There were also periods in which Kim was preoccupied with the obsession of hurting others, which led to her performing checking rituals and to her locking away knives and other sharp objects to prevent herself from acting on her obsessions.

DSM-IV Diagnoses

Axis I: 300.3   Obsessive-Compulsive Disorder
Axis II: 301.82   Avoidant Personality Disorder

Discussion

Kim's compulsive hoarding behavior justifies a diagnosis of OCD. This diagnosis is consistent with her past history of obsessions about harming others and with her accompanying checking rituals. The diagnostic picture is not complete, however, without accounting for Kim's pattern of avoidance and social isolation. A diagnosis of social phobia would seem to fit her fear of social situations in which she might be exposed to scrutiny by others, such as at social gatherings and in lines at the grocery store. However, the chronic, pervasive pattern of Kim's social isolation, her vulnerability to rejection, and her tendency to be overwhelmed by minor changes in her daily routine are better accounted for by the diagnosis of avoidant personality disorder. It is worth noting that Cluster C personality disorders, to which avoidant personality disorder belongs, are the most commonly reported personality disorders in patients with OCD.[1]

The interaction between OCD and other comorbid conditions is both fascinating and complex. Some personality disorders—especially those of Cluster C (i.e., dependent, passive-aggressive, avoidant, obsessive-compulsive)—may be a product of long-standing OCD. In Kim's case, one wonders how much of her avoidant personality disorder results from her inability to have anyone into her home other than close family members who know her "secret." One might also ask whether her avoidant personality disorder causes her to avoid interpersonal contact that might lead, in effect, to naturalistic behavior therapy, because she does not want to be faced with people entering her apartment.

Case Presentation 3
Destructive Compulsions

Kurt, 35 years of age, is currently an inpatient in a state mental hospital. He has been brought in for a reevaluation of his chronic

---

[1]Baer L, Jenike MA, Black DW, et al.: "Effect of Axis II Diagnoses on Treatment Outcome With Clomipramine in 55 Patients With Obsessive-Compulsive Disorder." *Archives of General Psychiatry* 49:862–866, 1992.

and extremely debilitating compulsive behaviors. He has been hospitalized because of the self-destructive nature of his compulsive behaviors, which include repeatedly putting his fingers into his mouth and pressing or pulling at his gums, lips, and jaw, causing ulcers and lacerations on his gums, buccal mucosa, and lips, as well as damage to his jaw. Recently, he has also begun to press on his eyes with his thumb to the point that staff members are worried about damage to his eyes. Kurt has no teeth; 5 years ago his symptoms were so severe that he removed most of his teeth, and the remainder were extracted because of abscesses caused by his pressing and battering his gums. Kurt says he is "obsessed" with his mouth and realizes that the urge to push or pull on it is crazy and bizarre but cannot stop himself from doing it. He feels a transient sense of relief after yielding to his destructive urges, but they soon reappear, sometimes within minutes. When he tries "to hold it in," his anxiety mounts and he finds it more and more difficult to control himself.

At present, management at the hospital of his case includes intermittently restraining him in a Gerri chair, which Kurt requests when he senses he is about to yield to his compulsions. He has been restrained in the chair for an average of 15 hours a week over the past several months.

During the interview, Kurt is initially able to restrain himself but later begins to pull at his mouth with gradually escalating frequency and vigor. He also displays tic-like movements of his toes and occasionally his hands and arms, and his voice tends to get loud when he becomes excited. Kurt is clearly agitated and desperate, saying that he is "not human" and that all he wants is to be "put to sleep like a dog."

Kurt's disorder first emerged at age 3 years, when he began to clap his hands repetitively and was noted to have a decreased attention span. He was described as "consistently bizarre" in his movements, which occasionally brought on teasing by peers. His condition was diagnosed as Tourette's disorder. At age 16 he experienced obsessions that someone might put ground glass in his food or that glass might get into his eyes. He also began to fear that he might strangle someone, started hoarding things under his rug, and became excessively meticulous about certain aspects of his room.

Before his current obsessions with his mouth developed, he engaged in another destructive ritual: moving his toes in his shoes repeatedly to the point that he blackened his toenails. Kurt managed to finish high school with support from his family, but he has never been able to hold a steady job and has been hospitalized for all but 6 weeks of the last 3 years. There is no history of Tourette's disorder or any other psychiatric problem in Kurt's family, with the exception of a suicide attempt by his brother.

DSM-IV Diagnoses

Axis I: 307.22   Chronic Motor or Vocal Tic Disorder
            300.3   Obsessive-Compulsive Disorder

Discussion

This case is an excellent example of the link between OCD and tic disorders. The patient is described as having long-standing Tourette's disorder, although the diagnosis of Tourette's requires multiple tics and one or more vocal tics. Because there are no vocal tics, the appropriate diagnosis may be chronic motor or vocal tic disorder. Kurt also meets the diagnostic criteria for OCD. His preoccupation with his mouth has an obsessive quality, he recognizes his behavior as senseless, and he desperately, albeit unsuccessfully, resists it. His self-destructive behavior is stereotyped and provides temporary relief from anxiety; moreover, he describes a history of typical obsessions and compulsions beginning in adolescence.

There is some phenomenological resemblance between OCD and tic disorders in the stereotyped, repetitive, and compulsive nature of the behavior. In addition, it has been shown that OCD bears a genetic relationship to Tourette's disorder. In a recent study, about 12% of the first-degree relatives of probands with Tourette's disorder had OCD, and the prevalence of current or past tic symptoms in patients with OCD was about 25%.[2]

[2]Pauls DL: "The Genetics of Obsessive Compulsive Disorder," in *Psychobiology of Obsessive Compulsive Disorder.* Edited by Zohar Y, Insel TR, Rasmussen SA. New

Finally, Kurt's condition has some similarity to Lesch-Nyhan syndrome, "a neurological syndrome comprising choreoathetosis, spasticity, a variable degree of mental deficiency, and a striking behavioural disturbance characterized by self-mutilation.[3] This syndrome occurs only in males, and the compulsive behavioral disturbance has its onset between the ages of 2 and 16 years. In Lesch-Nyhan syndrome, "episodes of involuntary and occasionally unilateral self-mutilation come and go without any clear relationship to endogenous or environmental factors" and are often associated with agitation or anxiety.[4] Lesch-Nyhan syndrome is caused by a severe deficiency in a particular enzyme, which results in marked overproduction of uric acid. In Kurt's case, uric acid levels were normal, making the diagnosis highly unlikely.

Case Presentation 4
The Shoplifter

Mary is a 55-year-old part-time retail salesperson in a large department store and the wife of a military retiree. She was referred for treatment of depression and obesity. Mary had symptoms and signs of dysthymia, including feelings of hopelessness and despair, crying spells, loss of energy, loss of interests, poor concentration, and compulsive eating. On further questioning, she reported a tendency to be a compulsive shopper; she had four credit cards and had run up all of them to the maximum amounts, putting the family under severe financial stress, as their only income sources were her husband's retirement compensation and her salary.

York, Springer-Verlag, 1990.

[3]Nuki G: "Disorders of Purine Metabolism," in *Oxford Textbook of Medicine.* Edited by Weatherall DJ, Ledingham JGG, Warrell DA. Oxford, UK, Oxford University Press, 1983, pp. 9.70–9.80; see p. 9.76.

[4]Op cit., p. 9.76.

Mary reported that her marriage has been unsatisfactory. Her husband, who suffers from diabetes and has had one leg amputated, is emotionally and physically disabled and spends almost all his time at home. The marital relationship has deteriorated to the point that husband and wife refuse to talk to each other and they try to get back at each other through passive-aggressive behavior.

Early in treatment, Mary had been encouraged to tear up her credit cards, which she did. However, she subsequently started shoplifting, which endangered her job at the department store.

During the course of psychotherapy, Mary reported having engaged in classic obsessive-compulsive behavior since her mid-teens, when a learning disability manifested. She was unable to distinguish between her right hand and her left, confused words, and was unable to separate *b* and *d* in her readings. The disorders caused her to spend hours reading a sentence or counting, followed by compulsive hand washing and showering in response to a fear of contamination, and later by constant checking of doors, light switches, burners, and garage doors. Along with these symptoms, she began hoarding, a symptom that has been progressive over the course of her adult life. She reports that she has not thrown anything away for many years. She has her papers, grades, and whatever friends have given her, dating from high school. In addition, she does not throw away newspapers, magazines, articles, pieces of clothing, or furniture, fearing that she might discard something of significance. Finally, she has developed various "collections," spending a great deal of money trying to add to them. Her garage is completely filled with newspapers, magazines, old kitchenware, furniture, and a variety of other objects. Three of her bedrooms and her living room are also filled with objects that she cannot throw away. Consequently, it is difficult for Mary and her husband to move freely about the house or do more than exist in the constricted space remaining.

Mary recognizes the irrationality of her hoarding, but she has no desire to rid herself of any of these objects for fear that she might need them some day. She even talks about passing objects along to her children rather than throwing them away.

DSM-IV Diagnoses

Axis I: 300.3   Obsessive-Compulsive Disorder
           312.32   Kleptomania
           300.4   Dysthymic Disorder
Axis II: 315.00   Reading Disorder
           (Developmental Reading Disorder)

Discussion

This case provides a good example of the interrelationship between OCD and the impulse-control disorders (intermittent explosive disorder, kleptomania, pathological gambling, pyromania, trichotillomania). Similarities between impulse-control disorders and OCD include 1) an inability to resist an impulse, drive, or temptation; and 2) an increasing sense of tension before committing the act. The impulse-control disorders differ from OCD in that 1) the act tends to be harmful to the person or others, and 2) the act is ego-syntonic—that is, pleasure or gratification is experienced at the time the act is performed. Some of these conditions (e.g., trichotillomania) are more closely identified with OCD than are others.

Mary's OCD dates from her high school years at least, and her symptoms are classic, including repeating, checking, washing, and hoarding. The learning disability is credible and clearly a contributory factor in her compulsive reading and counting. However, many patients describe diagnoses of dyslexia and resultant learning disabilities when, in fact, they have problems reading because of obsessional worry about understanding the material, which leads to compulsive rereading and, in turn, to their receiving the diagnosis of dyslexia or another learning disability.

A nuance of Mary's hoarding that should not go unnoticed is the tendency to pass objects on to her children for safekeeping and possible future use. This tendency suggests that she has completely filled her available storage space and is now encroaching on theirs. Her kleptomanic behavior may be a feature of the OCD as well, another aspect of Mary's need to hoard certain objects to decrease her obsessional anxiety or other feelings of discomfort. Typically, these patients feel that they may need the hoarded objects in the future and worry that harm will result if they discard them. In this instance there is the suggestion that Mary may have run up the bills on her credit cards to acquire objects for her hoard. Thus, when the cards were taken away, Mary was compelled to steal to decrease her obsessional anxiety. Finally, Mary's long-standing feelings of hopelessness and despair, and her crying spells, loss of energy, loss of interests, poor concentration, and compulsive eating, justify a diagnosis of dysthymic disorder.

Case Presentation 5
Shut Out of Her Home

Lisa was in her early 30s when she was first referred to the clinic. She was a skilled laboratory technician who was currently the head of a small, specialized section. During the initial visit, her immediate concern was about her marriage. This was Lisa's first marriage, which occurred after a short courtship soon after she had completed her technician's training. Within a few months, she and her husband had drifted apart. Her husband, also a professional, became increasingly immersed in his work. By the time of her visit, a few years had elapsed, and recognizing their differences, she and her husband were now separated and in the process of an amicable but inevitable divorce.

Lisa had long accepted some of the emotional consequences of the termination of her marriage. As the legal settlement neared, she knew that some emotional conflicts would crop up. Lisa had learned to depend on her husband for many household chores and financial matters. In addition, she believed that her parents would reject her divorce for emotional and religious reasons. They loved her husband and had no idea of the couple's mutual unhappiness.

Superficially it seemed that Lisa's concern about her parents' reaction had caused her anxiety and triggered her evaluation at the clinic. Short-term counseling through her employee's assistance program had not been helpful, and her anxiety symptoms were now interfering with her work.

At the initial interview she was extremely tense, restless, and often preoccupied; now she always seemed to anticipate the worst. By this time her husband had moved to his own apartment, and she was alone in their three-bedroom home. At work she felt fine, except for her lessened ability to concentrate. However, it was very difficult for her to feel at ease at home, and sleep was becoming a problem. Lisa now avoided social situations and crowds, and she felt frustrated about her continuing dependence on her husband for everyday things. At the time of the interview, Lisa was taking an H_2 receptor antagonist for a recurrence of long-quiescent gastrointestinal distress. She was often troubled by palpitations and tightness in her chest. She complained of fatigue and a variety of nonspecific muscular pains that were relieved by nonsteroidal anti-inflammatory drugs. In addition, her blood pressure was recently noted to be elevated, and she had begun treatment with an antihypertensive agent.

During the third interview some additional problems came into focus. Lisa shared the fact that during the last few weeks she had been living in a series of motels. In explaining her present living arrangements, she commented that no one, except for her husband, knew about certain symptoms that had emerged during her adolescence but had become more impairing after her marriage. Lisa had continuous, intense fears of contamination. Although her fears and the senseless cleaning and washing behavior her fears engendered would not bother her much at her work, they haunted her at home. She believed that everything in her home and all her personal belongings were contaminated by chemicals, disease, and pollution. Repeatedly cleaning these objects and washing herself no longer brought relief.

Lisa's concerns were principally about the health and safety of others and how she would act as a vehicle to transmit this "contamination." She had begun to "close" some of the rooms in her home because she felt they were hopelessly contaminated. First to be "closed," years ago, was the second bathroom, followed by the spare bedroom and many of the closets. As time progressed Lisa shut herself out of her home. Because her husband was no longer present to reassure her personally about the safety of certain objects and areas, she had made the decision to move out. However, she could remain at a motel for only 4 or 5 days because over time the motel room and its surroundings would also, Lisa felt, become contaminated. As her fascinating history unfolded, Lisa also disclosed that she was a "part-time" checker and hoarder and experienced episodes of compulsive hair pulling, the onset of which dated back to adolescence. These were the principal reasons that her marriage had failed.

DSM-IV Diagnoses

Axis I: 300.3   Obsessive-Compulsive Disorder
          309.24   Adjustment Disorder With Anxiety
          312.39   Trichotillomania

Discussion

Often patients with primary OCD will present with symptoms that suggest another psychiatric disorder. In Lisa's case, nonspecific anxiety symptoms were prominent, and the history of marital difficulties with separation and impending divorce warranted a diagnosis of adjustment disorder with anxiety. Although this diagnosis is accurate, it does not reflect the existence of underlying chronic and pervasive OCD, which precipitated, in large part, Lisa's marital difficulties that were the proximate cause of the adjustment disorder. Unless the clinician asks specific questions targeted to uncover obsessions and rituals, the diagnosis of OCD is often missed. General questions open the door to discussions of specific obsessions, compulsions, and rituals. For example, to initiate discussion of obsessions, the clinician might ask, "Do you have recurrent intrusive, unwanted thoughts, worries, images, or impulses that seem silly, nasty, or horrible?" For compulsions the clinician might ask, "Do you have behaviors like washing, checking, or tapping or mental behaviors involving counting or repeating a phrase that you feel compelled to do to lessen feelings of anxiety, discomfort, or disgust?"

In this case, the patient's OCD is clear. The onset of contamination fears in adolescence and resultant ritualistic cleaning of both herself and everything in her home are typical for patients with contamination obsessions. Her avoidance of entire rooms in her house may be viewed as extreme, but in fact many patients with contamination obsessions reach this extremity because of fear of both contamination and the price in hours or days they know they would pay if they were to begin a bout of cleaning/washing rituals. Lisa's fear that she will, indirectly of directly, contaminate others and cause contagion is common among OCD patients, although other patients may be fearful only of contamination causing illness or injury to themselves. Both kinds of obsessional fear can lead to extremes of avoidance of "contaminated" objects and to cleaning compulsions that can be incapacitating.

Interestingly, this case reveals a common but less frequently discussed component of OCD: the need for reassurance. Lisa's OCD worsened when her husband left, taking with him the reassurance that decreased her anxiety about being in her home. Reassurance rituals provide brief relief for persons with OCD but, predictably, become annoying to family members. As with other rituals, the reduction in anxiety reassurance rituals provide soon dissipates, and the person with OCD becomes addicted to reassurance, repeatedly requiring another "fix."

Case Presentation 6
Out of Kilter

Stanley is a 35-year-old married high school teacher who complains that he "can't stop obsessing." He is very hesitant, somewhat effem- inate in his manner, and tangential in describing his difficulties. He seems depressed and anxious, and frequently uses "I don't know," "you know," and "I guess" statements. Stanley's main obsession centers on what he should be doing with his life. He feels unable to make a commitment to his work or to his marriage. He describes himself as someone who has two personalities: the professional and "the bum." Deep inside, Stanley feels he is truly the bum. His professional career requires "acting"; it does not reflect his true, immature, incompetent self, which, according to Stanley, "doesn't really have the working knowledge to do the job." Stanley ruminates constantly about decisions he has made in the past and about decisions he is faced with presently. Should he, for example, become involved in community activities? Is this the right time for it? He is afraid that if he takes on this responsibility, he will be in "over his head" and arouse expectations he will be unable to meet. Stanley sometimes feels overwhelmed by the fear that he will not be able to "control the day." This is especially so if the day seems "glaring," "hard to see," or "different" when he wakes up in the morning; this signals to him that the rest of the day will be "out of kilter."

Stanley has experienced long periods of anxiety and depression. His wife, who has joined him for the interview, says that during these times he is especially dysfunctional, self-centered, and unavailable emotionally. Stanley's depression has typically been related to his belief that he is not functioning in his work the way he should. He has also always been anxious about how others view him: Do they see him as the professional or as the bum? He wants them to see him as the professional, but this would mean he would have to pretend to be somebody he really isn't. He has always feared that he would not be able to measure up to others' expectations and would make a commitment he would not be able to keep. Over the past 4 years he has seen two therapists, hoping that they could solve his problems. In the past month, he has felt changes in his "environment and personality" that are "scary . . . the overall look of things is different . . . focus is different . . . tints of colors are different." He feels he has finally developed the "working knowledge" of how to teach, through increased contact with his peers and help from his therapists, but he worries that he has given up his true self to make these changes.

DSM-IV Diagnoses

Axis I: 300.4   Dysthymic Disorder
Axis II: 301.9   Personality Disorder Not Otherwise Specified

Discussion

A diagnostic criterion for OCD requires the presence of either obsessions or compulsions. Stanley does not seem to have any compulsions. Obsessions, at least initially, must be experienced as intrusive and senseless, and the person must attempt to ignore, suppress, or neutralize them. In Stanley's case, these requirements are not met. His ruminations seem neither intrusive nor senseless to him, and there is no indication of any attempt to resist them. Stanley's ruminations may be related to his chronic low-level depression, as ruminations about the past, difficulty in making decisions, and low self-esteem are consistent with a diagnosis of dysthymic disorder. An alternative diagnosis would be mixed anxiety-depressive disorder if the anxiety and depressive symptoms were clinically meaningful yet did not meet criteria for a specific anxiety or mood disorder (classified in DSM-IV under "anxiety disorder not otherwise specified"). Stanley makes many statements suggesting symptoms of derealization, and some of his self statements might be viewed as symptoms of depersonalization. In addition, the unusual nature of his ruminations, the tangential and odd beliefs and verbalizations, and the excessive social anxiety justify a diagnosis of a mixed personality disorder with schizotypal, dependent, and obsessive-compulsive features.

CME Test
Chapter 1
Case Presentations 1–6

Please read the six sets of questions (12 questions total) that follow and circle the one best answer for each question on the corresponding answer sheet in the accompanying booklet.

Case Presentation 1: How Do I Know It Is Normal?

1A. Why is this case an atypical presentation of obsessive-compulsive disorder (OCD)?

1. It is accompanied by a major depression.
2. The patient is aware of, and disturbed by, his irresistible compulsion to reread X-ray films.
3. His compulsive behavior was triggered by a specific event occurring in his 30s.

1B. The patient's depression was considered secondary rather than primary. What was the basis of this diagnostic conclusion?

1. The patient had excessive guilt concerning his cousin's death.
2. His compulsive checking of X-ray films predated his dysphoric mood.
3. His relationship with his wife had deteriorated.

Case Presentation 2: The Wastebasket Apartment

2A. Why is the Axis II diagnosis in this case avoidant personality disorder rather than social phobia?

1. The patient is comfortable in some situations but not in others.
2. The patient is globally uncomfortable socially and depends heavily on certain persons for companionship.
3. The patient avoids having others see her sloppy apartment.

2B. The diagnosis of OCD is justified by which symptom(s)?

1. The patient's great difficulty in making decisions and her perception that nonroutine activities are overwhelmingly complex.
2. The patient's long history of social isolation and difficulties in interpersonal relationships.
3. The patient's irresistible urge to accumulate objects in her apartment.

Case Presentation 3: Destructive Compulsions

3A. The diagnosis of Tourette's disorder requires which of the following?

1. Multiple motor tics and one or more vocal tics
2. Either motor or vocal tics
3. Coprolalia

3B. This case demonstrates the high comorbidity of OCD and tic disorders. A current or past history of tic symptoms occurs in what percentage of patients with OCD?

1. 50%
2. 25%
3. 15%

Case Presentation 4: The Shoplifter

4A. The impulse-control disorder in this case is comorbid with OCD. What distinguishes impulse-control disorders from OCD?

1. A sense of pleasure other than relief of anxiety follows the act.
2. Anxiety is heightened by delay of the act.
3. Family life is often disrupted.

4B. What is an important distinction between dysthymic disorder and major depressive disorder?

1. Major depressive disorder is characterized by discrete episodes that can be distinguished from the person's usual functioning.

2. Dysthymic disorder is often associated with an Axis I disorder such as OCD.
3. Depressive symptoms are usually less severe in major depressive disorder than in dysthymic disorder.

Case Presentation 5: Shut Out of Her Home

5A. The patient's idea that she might be contaminating other people appears to have become nearly delusional. Why is the diagnosis in this case OCD rather than schizophrenia?

1. The obsession is recurrent, persistent, and irresistible.
2. The obsession gives rise to repetitive, purposeful behaviors.
3. The obsession is recognized by the patient as inappropriate.

5B. The patient's presenting symptoms appeared to reflect only adjustment disorder with anxiety. Why is the primary diagnosis OCD?

1. The symptoms of OCD had been present since adolescence but were masked before the marital separation.
2. The OCD symptoms led the patient to close herself out of her home and move to various motels, precipitating the adjustment disorder.
3. The adjustment disorder resulted from the marital separation and was totally unrelated to the OCD of many years' standing.

Case Presentation 6: Out of Kilter

6A. This patient has a preoccupation that he is not functioning as a professional in his work and that he could not possibly measure up to the expectations of others. Why does this symptom picture not qualify for a diagnosis of OCD?

1. The preoccupation is not experienced as intrusive or senseless by the patient, who does not attempt to resist it.
2. The preoccupation is based on reality, e.g., a long history of professional failure.
3. The preoccupation has not interfered with the patient's actual functioning as a professional.

6B. What justifies the secondary diagnosis of personality disorder not otherwise specified in this case?

1. The patient's obsessions are related to chronic low-level depression.
2. Excessive social anxiety, together with schizotypal, dependent, and obsessive-compulsive features, is present.
3. The patient perceives himself as pretending to be someone he is not.

Case Presentation 7
Multiple Complaints

Ann, a 44-year-old married mother of two, complains of feelings of depression and anxiety, which have worsened recently. She cries easily, finds it hard to break out of feelings of sadness and hopelessness, and does not enjoy the company of others. She falls asleep easily but then wakes up in the middle of the night, unable to continue her sleep. Most of the time she has no appetite, but at other times she compulsively binges on snacks. Her worst feelings are in the morning hours, when she cannot find the energy to get up and get going. Ann is also hampered by severe fear of contamination and of causing harm to others. She has multiple compulsions, mostly related to her fear of contamination. She washes her hands at least 15 times a day, always soaping them three or four times. In doing her laundry, she must use the "perfect amount" of detergent and later must clean the washing machine with disinfectant. She cannot sit on a bed, even in her own home, and will not use a public toilet other than in a hospital or a hotel. In addition, Ann has lately experienced what seem to be full-blown panic attacks, and now she will not drive outside of town unaccompanied, for fear that she will panic and "lose control."

Ann's symptoms of anxiety and depression started 20 years ago during a period of marital discord and family problems. She had difficulty sleeping, gained weight as a result of compulsive bingeing, and developed a variety of phobias, including one involving fire. She has been hospitalized for depression several times over the years and received electroconvulsive therapy. A few days after the birth of her second child, 16 years ago, she suddenly developed a fear of harming the child and became severely depressed. Her fear of contamination and compulsive rituals started 5 years later, and several years of psychodynamic therapy have not helped her overcome them.

Psychiatric problems are common in Ann's family. Her younger sister is depressed and exhibits compulsive hoarding behaviors, and her daughter has bulimia. Two of her brothers have been treated for paranoia, and all her brothers use alcohol excessively.

DSM-IV Diagnoses

Axis I   296.32   Major Depressive Disorder, Recurrent, Moderate
          300.3   Obsessive-Compulsive Disorder
          300.21   Panic Disorder With Agoraphobia

Discussion

Ann presents a complex picture of multiple and chronic symptoms of depression and anxiety. Her current symptoms meet the criteria for major depression, and Ann's history indicates a recurrent pattern. Her obsessions and rituals justify a diagnosis of obsessive-compulsive disorder (OCD). Finally, her recent panic attacks, leading to the inability to drive out of town, satisfy the criteria for panic disorder with agoraphobia. Identifiable precipitants for OCD onset occur in less than 30% of cases. When they do occur, they often involve some aspect of childbearing, including infertility, pregnancy, delivery, caring for a newborn, or abortion (either spontaneous or therapeutic). As in Ann's case, comorbid conditions (in this instance depression) sometimes predate the onset of OCD by several years. The combination of depression and OCD is common: about 75% of patients with OCD have symptoms of depression when their disorder is first diagnosed, and about 30% have major depression. In most cases the depression is secondary, developing after the onset of OCD. In Ann's case, however, the depression seems by history to be primary. Frequently, as in this case, there is a tendency for obsessive-compulsive symptoms to worsen in conjunction with worsening of comorbid conditions. The comorbidity of panic disorder and OCD, also seen in this case, is less common than that of OCD and depression. It is found in only about 10% of patients with OCD, but this is more than 10 times the rate of panic disorder in the population without OCD.

Case Presentation 8
A Nervous Wreck

Donna is a 33-year-old woman who appears distraught, crying often as she tells her story to the psychiatrist. Nine years ago, when she worked as a dental hygienist, she experienced what she later learned were panic attacks. She felt that these attacks were always associated with the presence of certain patients and not others; she would become anxious when anticipating having to work with those patients with whom she associated the onset of panic. A year later she had a panic attack while driving with her sister on the highway. As a result, she began to avoid driving on the highway in the company of others. Various other stressors, such as talking to her boss or to others in positions of authority, also seemed to trigger panic attacks. Donna found herself developing rituals, such as shaking items of clothing a certain number of times before putting them away or wrapping up disposable diapers a particular number of times before throwing them in the trash bin. She felt that these rituals would somehow ward off the intensely feared panic attacks.

Donna's compulsive rituals worsened considerably 6 months ago, when she developed a habit of filling out her baby book after visits with the pediatrician. She was compelled to rewrite entire pages of the book if something went wrong during the writing process. For example, a red mark on the page would remind her of blood; writing over a black or gray dot on the page would make her think that cancer would strike her child. In both instances she would have to write the page over again to protect her child. Donna felt desperate when she "couldn't keep up" with her rituals. She lost her appetite and became severely depressed and suicidal. She asked her husband to take over the writing in the baby book, but this provided no relief. Since initiating treatment, Donna has continued to develop an ever-increasing number of checking and counting rituals, spending several hours of each day and night preoccupied with these tasks. If she sees something shiny while driving, she is compelled to backtrack and check it. If she sees a word on a sign, she must return and check whether the dot in the letter "i" is round or square. She is compelled to remove lint from clothes and to cut off all the dots when clipping coupons. She rinses things out before throwing them away. She repeats certain behaviors, such as turning the dryer on and off, climbing upstairs repeatedly with particular types of laundry items, and shaking the blankets 6 or 12 times. Most of the rituals are intended to ward off panic attacks or to protect her children, though she is well aware that "it's totally crazy." She describes herself in her present condition as a "nervous wreck" and feels that she can blame only herself for her problems.

DSM-IV Diagnoses

Axis I: 300.21   Panic Disorder With Agoraphobia
           300.3   Obsessive-Compulsive Disorder
           296.2x   Major Depressive Disorder, Single Episode

Discussion

This case illustrates an interesting chronological development of several mental disorders. It appears that Donna's current difficulties were originally triggered by the terrifying experience of panic attacks. In an attempt to cope with the threat of panic attacks, she developed "prevention tactics," including avoiding driving in the company of others and creating a series of "superstitious" rituals. It should be noted that Donna's avoidance of driving with other people is atypical, because panic attack patients most commonly prefer to drive in the company of another person (as in Case Presentation 7). More and more rituals developed over time, particularly as Donna attempted to cope with the anxiety-provoking thoughts of harm to her children. Also, as is typical with patients with OCD who are married, she soon enmeshed her husband in the illness process by asking him to take over writing in the baby book. Eventually, her inability to keep up with her increasing repertoire of "protective" rituals led to depression. The chronological development in the patient of multiple disorders is not uncommon in OCD patients. The case is also a good example of the difference between DSM-III and DSM-III-R in that the latter eliminated diagnostic hierarchies and allowed the use of multiple diagnoses, without asserting the order of focus of attention or treatment. This convention is continued in DSM-IV.

Case Presentation 9
Losing Weight

Anthony is a thin, athletic-looking 18-year-old high school graduate who appears fatigued and worried and is markedly hesitant in his speech. According to his mother and sister, who brought him to the interview, Anthony has a history of minor rituals dating back to grammar school. They remember his touching the door in a particular way while closing it and engaging in bathroom rituals involving toothbrushing and showering. These compulsive behaviors, however, were not of such magnitude that they significantly interfered with his functioning. In addition, Anthony describes himself as having a long-standing tendency to seek the input of others and to follow their example in determining his own actions. He also says he has always been concerned about being overweight (he is 5'9" and has weighed 210 pounds most of his adult life), but his previous attempts to lose weight had not been successful.

Anthony's father died of lung cancer 5 months ago, just 6 weeks after the malignancy had been diagnosed. Soon after his father's death, Anthony became very rigorous in his pursuit of weight loss. Since then he has been following a highly structured routine: He arises each morning early enough to watch the sun rise. He eats a breakfast consisting of 1 ounce of cereal, one-half cup of skim milk, one hard-boiled egg, and strawberries or blueberries. He then waits a short period of time before proceeding to the weight room, where, from Monday through Friday, he spends almost exactly 2 hours performing an identical routine of weight lifting, unless someone else is there, which permits him to break his routine by following another's. He skips lunch (today was an exception, because his mother "forced" him to have it) and has a supper consisting of a sandwich, 6 ounces of yogurt, and iced tea. He does eat salads at times but is concerned about possible ill effects from pesticides that might have been applied to the vegetables. As a result of this ritualized regimen over the past several months, Anthony has lost 75 pounds, reportedly stabilizing his weight at 135 pounds about 2 weeks ago. Anthony says he would prefer to weigh 145 pounds, which would be appropriate for his height, but is unable to eat the foods that would allow him to gain weight. Recently, he has expressed an interest in pursuing a career as a dietitian.

Other rituals have also increased considerably since Anthony's father's death. Washing, dressing, and cleaning now involve complex and rigid routines, and Anthony becomes quite anxious if his routine is interrupted. He is very concerned about his physical well-being and often checks his appearance in the mirror. He also has a lengthy daily routine of checking the lawn in the backyard of his house. In addition, he is very indecisive, seeking reassurance and advice from family members before taking even minor actions such as choosing clothes to wear.

DSM-IV Diagnosis

Axis I: 300.3   Obsessive-Compulsive Disorder

Discussion

The combination of an eating disorder with OCD is fairly common. Many patients with primary eating disorders, particularly anorexic patients, have obsessions about food and attendant compulsive eating rituals; moreover, in a sizable percentage of cases, patients with eating disorders also have OCD. For patients with primary OCD, there also have been reports of concurrent or past eating disorders. (In one study, 11% of women with OCD reported a history of anorexia.[1]) In Anthony's case, however, OCD alone seems to be the correct diagnosis. He has had rituals dating back to childhood, and his recent excessive effort to lose weight is embedded in a wide-ranging exacerbation of obsessive and compulsive symptoms. In this regard, it is important to note that the death of Anthony's father appears to have been the stressor that allowed scattered obsessive-compulsive symptoms and signs to coalesce into a disorder. Before the death of his father, Anthony did not meet criterion C for DSM-IV OCD because the obsessions and compulsions were neither markedly distressing nor sufficiently time-consuming to interfere significantly with his life. In terms of his eating problem, because Anthony has not lost enough weight to be considered anorexic and because he does not binge or purge, a secondary diagnosis of eating disorder not otherwise specified is not warranted at this time.

Case Presentation 10
The Man With Hypochondriacal Complaints

Neil was a certified public accountant working for a small but distinguished firm in a large city. He was referred by an otolaryngologist for evaluation of an "overwhelming anxiety with a phobia that he had cancer of the nose and throat." Careful evaluation of his symptoms did not uncover any tissue abnormalities.

At the time of his first visit, Neil described spending hours in the bathroom clearing his throat and vomiting to see whether there was blood in his throat. His fear that he had cancer was indeed overwhelming. During successive sessions he would ask at least 50 to 60 times whether he had cancer. He would check both hands and, upon

[1]Fahy TA, Osacar A, Marks I: "History of Eating Disorders in Female Patients With Obsessive-Compulsive Disorder." *International Journal of Eating Disorders* 14:439–443, 1993.

finding that his left hand was slightly different from the right, would ask whether cancer caused this difference. Reassurance did not help; it simply led to another question. A casual comment by the therapist such as "I'm pretty sure you are OK" would lead Neil to conclude, "Well, then you really do think I have cancer."

After 2 years, Neil left therapy and was not seen again until 5 years later, when, once again, he became terrified that he was living with cancer. This second instance was apparently the result of his having had a routine physical examination in which urinalysis showed several red blood cells. The conclusion was that the hematuria was idiopathic and benign. Neil refused to accept this diagnosis. He led the doctor on by asking the generic question "What are the possible causes of red blood cells in the urine?" The doctor, not recognizing Neil's terror, stated that it could be one of numerous things, including cancer. This remark threw Neil into a panic, and he returned to therapy.

Psychotherapy continued on a regular basis for 2 years. At this point, Neil's condition took a turn for the worse as a result of the following incident: One night while he was having dinner in a restaurant, Neil went to the men's room. Upon finding that there were no more fresh towels on which to dry his hands, he used a towel that was in the wastebasket. On the way out of the restaurant, he began to wonder whether the person who had used the towel before him had acquired immunodeficiency syndrome (AIDS). He then developed an obsessional fear of AIDS that utterly overwhelmed his previous fears of cancer.

In a matter of months, the fear of AIDS drove Neil to the point that he could stand the tension no longer and admitted himself to a local psychiatric hospital. Shortly afterward, he moved to a large, well-known hospital in another metropolitan area. There, the diagnosis of OCD was made and specific treatment begun.

DSM-IV Diagnoses

Axis I: 300.7   Hypochondriasis vs.
           297.1   Delusional Disorder, Somatic Type vs.
           300.3   Obsessive-Compulsive Disorder

Discussion

The case presents an interesting differential diagnosis, which includes hypochondriasis; and delusional disorder, somatic type; and OCD. The patient certainly meets DSM-IV criteria A and B for hypochondriasis: "preoccupation with fears of having, or the idea that one has, a serious disease" that "persists despite appropriate medical evaluation and reassurance."[2] The question is whether in Neil's case the belief of having an illness is of delusional intensity; that is, can he acknowledge the possibility that his fears of having, or the idea that he has, a serious disease is unfounded? In addition, the case is a good example of the interrelationship of both hypochondriasis and delusional disorder with OCD. Neil also meets the DSM-IV criteria for OCD, with obsessions of a somatic nature. The pathological doubting and the need for constant reassurance he exhibits during therapy are especially characteristic of the patient with OCD. Poor insight may develop during the course of OCD. Although this degree of distress and this intensity of fears border on the delusional, OCD is not excluded by the patient's poor insight. Given the limitations of the information presented in the case history and given the diagnostic overlap, all three diagnoses must be cited. Finally, one wonders whether the 5-year hiatus in therapy represented a period of remission or whether the patient remained out of treatment but was still obsessed with having cancer.

Case Presentation 11
A Problem of Church and State

Louise, a 57-year-old married mother of six, has been in treatment with various psychiatrists for a period of 20 years. Treatment was

[2]American Psychiatric Association: *Diagnostic and Statistical Manual of Mental Disorders*, 4th Edition. Washington, D.C., American Psychiatric Association, 1994, p. 465.

initiated following a death in the family. At that time the patient suffered a panic attack, manifested by a racing heart, trembling, sweating, lightheadedness, and feelings of being in another world followed by anxiety, inability to sleep, and general restlessness. Symptoms of anxiety and depression, together with feelings of helplessness and social withdrawal, have persisted over the years.

At the time of the initial panic attack, the patient reports having told her obsessive thoughts to a psychiatrist, who informed her that these symptoms were persistent, very difficult to treat, and likely to be with her during the remainder of her life. Louise left this psychiatrist because of his "negative attitude."

The patient had attended Catholic schools in which disciplinary codes were rigidly enforced. She remained tense throughout her schooling and felt guilty about many deeds, especially a single instance of sexual play with a child approximately 3½ years old when Louise was about 8 years of age. Other examples of having sinned included eating a piece of cake before receiving Communion and being preoccupied with sinful thoughts.

Nineteen years into treatment, the patient reported that she was having increased difficulty with feelings of guilt arising from the fact that her husband worked in a hospital sterilizing instruments used in abortions. In fact, Louise was so disturbed, she wanted her husband to quit his job.

Further discussions have revealed that Louise continues to have obsessive thoughts of molesting a child. She reports strong guilty feelings for having such thoughts. Compulsive behavior is exhibited in the requirements that her Bible be placed in a particular place and that its corners be directed at specific angles. Louise feels compelled to continually see that the Bible remains in this position and that it is dusted frequently.

Louise's guilty feelings extend to other aspects of her life. She is so afraid of being accused of shoplifting that when she makes purchases she must check the shopping bag frequently to be sure no other items are in it. Even after she returns to the safety of her home, she must verify that the items are correctly noted on the receipt.

Of the patient's six children, two are reported to suffer from panic disorder to the extent that they are under psychological and pharmacological therapy.

DSM-IV Diagnoses

Axis I: 300.3   Obsessive-Compulsive Disorder
           300.21   Panic Disorder With Agoraphobia, Probable
                     (not a focus of treatment)

Discussion

This patient clearly meets the criteria for OCD, having long-standing obsessions with "sin" involving sexual behaviors, failures in Communion practices (be they rules of her own making or codified within Catholicism), and shoplifting; her rituals include straightening, dusting, and checking her Bible as well as checking her purchases and repeatedly asking her husband to change his job. Although her actions might be seen merely as aspects of her being a highly religious person, her religious beliefs, dominated as they are by recurrent thoughts of sinning, cause distress and dysfunction rather than providing solace. Such preoccupation with religious ideas and practices has been recognized by the Catholic Church for several hundred years as *scrupulosity*. OCD may occur more frequently in persons raised in any religion with strong proscription of certain behaviors and frequent ritualistic practices.

It is unclear whether the initial anxiety for which the patient sought treatment was associated with a panic attack or was part of an adjustment disorder with anxious features occurring in the wake of a family member's death. Panic disorder is comorbid with OCD in up to 10% of OCD patients, a rate more than 10 times greater than that in the population at large. Although Louise has had symptoms of other anxiety disorders over time that have been the focus of treatment in the past, her current complaints and problems center on obsessions, compulsions, and rituals and their effects on her life.

The presence of clinically significant panic disorder in two of the patient's six children points toward a probable diagnosis of panic disorder in the mother, as the prevalence of panic disorder is high in other family members with this condition.

Case Presentation 12
Bad People

Stephanie is a 16-year-old who should have been starting her junior year of high school. She had missed the spring semester of her sophomore year and refused to return to school because of the "bad people" she would encounter there.

In sixth grade, Stephanie had heavily invested herself in religion and daily prayer even though her family did not attend church on a regular basis. Within a year, this "preoccupation" faded, and Stephanie had good seventh- and eighth-grade years. Over the summer before entering high school, Stephanie seemed unusually "serious and distracted," and, in retrospect, her parents realized she had lost weight. When they began to observe her eating habits, they found she often ate very slowly, chewed her food deliberately, and would sometimes spit out food. Stephanie's pediatrician was concerned about an eating disorder, and when Stephanie's weight fell more than 15%, he referred her to an eating disorders specialist. Stephanie had never purged with vomiting, laxatives, or diuretics and could not or would not explain her eating behaviors. Individual and family therapy sessions yielded only a grudging acknowledgment that she was troubled by "bad people" and raised concern that schizophrenia might be emerging.

Psychotherapy continued through her freshman and sophomore years because Stephanie had more and more difficulty with both academic work and social relationships, neither of which had been problems before. By the spring of her sophomore year, she seemed unable to do schoolwork, was clearly depressed, and exhibited behaviors that seemed, in a word, bizarre. In addition to her eating behaviors, Stephanie seemed blocked when reading. She bought and discarded pencils at an "incredible" rate, refused to sleep in her room or to sit on certain pieces of furniture, and "camped out" on one sofa, asking others not to use it. Her obvious distress and dysfunction at school and with her family and friends failed to yield to individual and family psychotherapy, and it was unclear what her diagnosis was. It was suggested that Stephanie be sent to a renowned hospital for long-term, intensive inpatient treatment. Because the prescribed treatment was beyond the family's means, Stephanie and her family were referred instead for consultation.

In response to the usual questionnaires sent by the clinic before the intake session, Stephanie bluntly disclosed the following: "When I see people who I think use drugs or marijuana, they usually don't bother me until after I am away from them. Then I get their images in my mind, and feel that they are bad, unclean, unhealthy, and disgusting. I'm afraid they will make the world in my mind all dark and polluted, so I replace the "bad people" with "good people." When I am near the bad people for a long time (as in school), their effect on my mind seems more powerful. I have trouble doing any actions with the "bad people" in my head. This includes such things as eating, bathing, dressing, writing, reading, and playing the clarinet. I'm afraid to name my bad people (out loud) or describe the bad parts of my thoughts."

When seen with her family, Stephanie has great difficulty describing these thoughts, because expressing them in front of others seems to intensify her distress. At this initial interview, Stephanie looks sad and acknowledges "depression" both over feeling "crazy" and over the loss of friends and functioning that resulted from her preoccupation with "bad people." In private, later, she discloses that bad people use drugs, swear, shoplift, vandalize, tease, cheat, fuss, or are simply "too loud." At times, her distress over these "bad people" would become so extreme that she would either freeze in her tracks or want to scream or run away. She notes that at these times her heart beat unusually rapidly and forcefully, she felt that she could not get her breath, and she broke into a sweat.

DSM-IV Diagnosis

Axis I: 300.3   Obsessive-Compulsive Disorder

Discussion

In one sense, Stephanie's OCD symptoms first emerged in the form of unusual religiosity, but this harbinger of OCD would not satisfy the criteria for that diagnosis because it did not interfere with Stephanie's functioning or cause distress. At age 14, her preoccupation with "bad people" began. She tried to balance "bad people" with "good people" in a sort of double-entry bookkeeping system. However, many "good people" crossed over to the "bad people" side of Stephanie's ledger when they transgressed her strict behavioral boundaries. She interrupted any activity (e.g., eating, bathing, reading, writing) if obsessions about "bad people" intruded, and this avoidance ritual explained many of her seemingly bizarre behaviors. Thus, she could not swallow food she was chewing if the thought of a bad person intervened. Similarly, pencils she was using when thoughts of bad people invaded her consciousness became "infested" or "contaminated" and had to be discarded. She avoided sleeping in her bed for fear that it would become infested, and avoided sitting on certain chairs in her house that had been "contaminated" by "bad people" who had sat in them. By asking others to stay away from the sofa on which she sat and slept, she was able to protect it from possible "contamination." Her anxiety in this regard arose from the fact that she could never be certain whether anyone who might sit there had ever uttered an obscenity or used an illicit substance. Other rituals involved people's names and the number of letters in their names.

The intensity and near-delusional quality of her obsessions were alarming, but she retained some insight into the falsity of these beliefs and a strong sense that she was the only one who struggled with them. This sense of solitary "craziness" also kept her from disclosing her thoughts.

Although Stephanie clearly experienced panic attacks, they occurred only in the context of obsessional anxiety. The panic attacks increased her distress, but they were never a specific concern, and their severity paled in comparison with her obsessional torment. She described herself as "depressed," but she denied vegetative symptoms of depression and was most "depressed" about the interference with her functioning and the specific distress caused by her obsessions and rituals. She continued to like the taste of the food she succeeded in eating, slept soundly, and described having adequate energy if she was not interrupted by an obsession. She had no thoughts of suicide. An eating disorder was not present, because the patient thought herself too thin and abnormal eating behaviors developed only in association with her primary obsessional fear of "bad people" and without regard to issues of weight, thinness, or calories.

CME Test
Chapter 2
Case Presentations 7–12

Please read the six sets of questions (12 questions total) that follow and circle the one best answer for each question on the corresponding answer sheet in the accompanying booklet.

Case Presentation 7: Multiple Complaints

7A. Comorbidity of depression and obsessive-compulsive disorder (OCD) is common. What factor makes this case of such comorbidity unusual?

1. The additional diagnosis of panic disorder occurs together with the other two diagnoses.
2. Severe depression was triggered by the birth of a child.
3. The depression is primary rather than secondary.

7B. The onset of OCD in this case may have been associated with obsessions about contamination that developed a few years after the birth of a child. Identifiable precipitants for OCD occur in what percentage of cases?

1. >70%
2. <30%
3. 50%

Case Presentation 8: A Nervous Wreck

8A. In many cases of OCD, rituals are associated with a specific purpose. What is different about the functions of this patient's rituals early in the course of her OCD?

1. The early rituals were associated with writing in her baby books.
2. The early rituals were designed to ward off panic attacks.
3. The early rituals led to panic attacks.

8B. What important difference between DSM-III and DSM-IV is illustrated by this case presentation?

  1. DSM-IV has broadened definitions of some disorders to reflect new research findings.
  2. DSM-IV focuses on etiology and pathophysiology of mental disorders.
  3. DSM-IV has eliminated many diagnostic hierarchies and allows the use of multiple diagnoses.

Case Presentation 9: Losing Weight

9A. The patient in this case has elaborate and rigid eating rituals, and he has lost 75 pounds and wants to lose more. Why is an additional DSM-IV diagnosis of eating disorder not otherwise specified or of anorexia nervosa not made?

  1. The patient has not lost sufficient weight to meet the criteria for anorexia nervosa, and he does not binge or purge.
  2. The patient bases his actions on the opinions of others.
  3. Primary OCD is associated with eating disorders in only 12% of patients.

9B. What factor differentiates this patient's history of "minor rituals" observed since childhood from the full-blown OCD diagnosed at age 18?

  1. The patient's highly structured eating and exercise routines.
  2. The magnitude of the present symptoms, which are distressing and time-consuming.
  3. The patient's obsessive concern with seeking the opinion of others before taking action.

Case Presentation 10: The Man With Hypochondriacal Complaints

10A. In this case, what is the DSM-IV criterion for diagnosing delusional disorder, somatic type?

  1. The patient's inability to consider the possibility that the feared disease may not, in fact, be present.

2. The patient's tendency to manipulate physicians into stating that certain signs, such as red blood cells in the urine, could be associated with cancer.
3. The patient's overwhelming phobia about cancer and, later, about AIDS.

10B. What fact of this case is especially characteristic of the patient with OCD?

1. The patient's overwhelming fear of having cancer.
2. The patient's pathological doubting and need for constant reassurance.
3. The patient's excessive vomiting to determine whether there is blood in his throat.

Case Presentation 11: A Problem of Church and State

11A. What reinforces the diagnosis of probable panic disorder in this case?

1. Two of the patient's six children also suffer from clinically significant panic disorder.
2. The patient is uncomfortable when she goes out shopping.
3. Comorbidity of panic disorder and OCD is very common.

11B. What justifies diagnosing OCD in this case rather than seeing the patient as simply an excessively religious person?

1. The patient's extreme guilt about the nature of her husband's job and her "sinful" thoughts.
2. Her fear of being accused of shoplifting.
3. The distressing and dysfunctional effect of her guilt-provoking thoughts.

Case Presentation 12: Bad People

12A. This patient describes episodes of sweating, rapid heartbeat, and difficulty getting her breath. Why is panic disorder not a diagnosis in this case?

1. There is an insufficient number of symptoms to justify the diagnosis.

    2. The attacks were triggered by an identifiable obsessional stimulus.

    3. The patient was not disturbed by the symptoms.

12B. The differential diagnosis of this case was initially difficult; for example, the patient's eating behavior suggested an eating disorder. What factor finally led to a single diagnosis of OCD?

    1. The patient had developed bizarre rituals in addition to the unusual eating behaviors.

    2. Extreme religiosity in junior high school predicted the eventual development of OCD.

    3. The eating behavior was triggered by thoughts of "bad people."

Case Presentation 13
A Counting Nightmare

Jean, who is in her late 40s, describes herself as a valued paralegal for a major law firm. Her ambition had been to become an attorney; however, she gave up this goal because she had been troubled since early adolescence by obsessions with numbers, and compulsions, which consisted almost exclusively of counting. She also reports some depressive symptoms, principally resulting from her compulsive disorder and some ongoing family problems. Jean is not particularly anxious during the initial interview. She explains that her compulsive symptoms have been continuous, and there does not seem to be a particular stressor to explain their emergence.

Jean is divorced and now lives alone. She is generally in good health, and there is no history of present or past substance abuse. In addition, there is no history of medical or psychiatric intervention for her presenting complaint. In fact, she explains that until now, no one knew about her "counting" except her daughter.

Jean's eye contact, response time, continuity of thought, and attentiveness are excellent during the interview. It is difficult to understand what she means by "counting," yet she assures the interviewer that it is happening even as she speaks. When Jean is asked to give an example of her symptoms, her distress becomes obvious: "Doctor, I count everything, everywhere . . . whenever I see things in a series, I feel that I need to know *exactly* how many there are." When asked for a specific example, after briefly hesitating, she points at the wall and says, "I know how many diplomas are there." She has been directly facing the wall during the short interview, and it seems to the interviewer that counting the number of diplomas is not such a difficult task. Before this observation could be interjected, however, she continues: "I also know how many acoustic tiles are on the ceiling, how many slats there are in the vertical blinds on the windows, and how many stripes there are on your shirt. At the moment, I am working on counting the books on the top shelf over there."

The interview has progressed very smoothly, so naturally the question arises as to whether she really can do this. When asked how many stripes are on the interviewer's shirt, she responds correctly, adding, "And I am almost through with the top bookshelf." When tested on the vertical blinds, she is again correct. When Jean is pressed for an explanation, it becomes obvious that there are no "magical" methods to her counting. Her need is to know the exact number and to remember it for as long as possible. As she puts it, "After I count something once, I have to count it again and again until I am sure the number is right." There is no question that Jean's compulsion to count all the things around her is extremely thorough, but at the same time it is very disruptive and disturbing.

DSM-IV Diagnosis

Axis I: 300.3   Obsessive-Compulsive Disorder

Discussion

Jean's condition clearly meets the criteria for obsessive-compulsive disorder (OCD). The patient has a long history of an obsessional need to know the numbers of things in her environment, which leads to endless compulsive counting and checking rituals. She is compelled to check and recheck the number of things she has already counted to reassure herself that the totals are correct. It is interesting to note that compulsions (rituals) can be entirely mental, as in Jean's case. A distinction between obsessions and mental compulsions is that the former tend to be anxiogenic (i.e., raise anxiety), whereas the latter are anxiolytic (i.e., relieve or reduce anxiety). Recognition of purely mental compulsions was first formalized in DSM-IV.

Another interesting aspect of Jean's case is that although she realizes that her obsession with numbers is intrusive and senseless and the counting compulsions are irrational and distracting, she derives a certain feeling of superiority from her symptoms. She knows that her abilities are unusual, and she has a distorted sense of satisfaction and accomplishment as a result of her behavior. The depressive symptoms that Jean reports fall short of satisfying the DSM-IV criteria for major depressive disorder or dysthymic disorder.

Perhaps the most amazing feature of this case is the interference that Jean has had in life because of OCD. In spite of her rituals, Jean carries a greater percentage of the workload in her office than do her co-workers and is totally reliable, thorough, punctual, and very well organized.

Case Presentation 14
A Diagnostic Dilemma

Alvin is a semiretired businessman who had been quite successful and is currently able to maintain a comfortable lifestyle from his investment income alone. He is in his late 40s, divorced, and living alone. His only regular family contacts are with his mother and his children. They seem very close, but Alvin has little interaction with others in his extended family, and he has few friends. Alvin has never before consulted a mental health professional and is markedly anxious at the start of the interview.

Twenty minutes into the initial session, Alvin is asked to disclose his symptoms. After briefly hesitating, he removes his eyeglasses, points at his eyes, and says, "Come on, Doctor, I know you are just trying to be kind." Alvin has no eyebrows or eyelashes, and, indeed, after he points this fact out, their absence becomes obvious. On the other hand, he has a very light complexion, is becoming bald, and wears large glasses with thick lenses and wide frames that disguise his condition. Alvin's predominant mood during the interview is not that of passive embarrassment, as with most patients with OCD or trichotillomania, but anger—anger at himself for his irrational compulsion, and anger and frustration at the interviewing clinician for "knowing" about his condition but not confronting him with it.

Alvin agrees to participate in a medication research study during the next several months. Conjointly, he is invited to attend a support group. He is relatively quiet during his first support group meeting but manages to monopolize essentially all the group's time during the next meeting that he attends. Soon after the meeting starts, Alvin accosts the other group members with the following: "I know some of you are wondering why I am here, but I know that most of you know!" It was the "You can tell!" routine once again, but this time with the group. After his proclamation, he dramatically removes his glasses. Members of the group quickly confront him with the obvious facts: that his fair complexion, eyeglasses, and receding hair had disguised his condition. Alvin is not satisfied. He sees himself as a grossly disfigured monster who is in effect walking around with a sign across his chest reading, "Yes, I pull out my eyebrows and eyelashes . . . I have OCD . . . so what!"

Reanalysis of Alvin's disorder reveals that although there is no doubt about his compulsive hair pulling, his atypical reaction during the initial interview raises questions about his diagnosis. Is the compulsive hair pulling more an act of self-mutilation in a person with basically a histrionic or paranoid personality or dysmorphophobia, or is it symptomatic of an impulse-control disorder, specifically trichotillomania? During his next appointment, it becomes apparent that Alvin's belief that "everybody knows" is almost delusional: "My barber knows, my optometrist knows, my doctor [his primary care physician] knows . . . everyone knows and stares . . . but they are just too polite to say anything about it."

To the surprise of the group, Alvin begins to improve. There is an underlying depressive mood to his anger, which becomes evident after a few visits and which responds decisively to medication. In addition, he becomes less anxious, and with time, he reluctantly admits that perhaps members of the group and others "did not know." He is certainly pulling out hair with less and less frequency, and as the weeks pass, he proudly would show an individual hair or a cluster of "fuzz" that he spared. He is greatly relieved that he can now resist some of the impulses to pull.

DSM-IV Diagnoses

Axis I: 312.39   Trichotillomania
           300.7   Body Dysmorphic Disorder (Dysmorphophobia)

Discussion

A number of conditions appear to be closely associated with OCD. These conditions, termed obsessive-compulsive "variants" or "obsessive-compulsive spectrum disorders," include trichotillomania, nail biting, body dysmorphic disorder (dysmorphophobia), depersonalization disorder, somatization disorder, delusional disorder (somatic type), posttraumatic stress disorder, and eating disorders. In addition to these conditions, the line between "typical" compulsions and impulse-control disorders such as (compulsive) drinking, smoking, gambling, eating, shopping, or stealing (kleptomania) can be very thin.

Among the obsessive-compulsive variants, trichotillomania (i.e., compulsive hair pulling) has recently been discovered to be more common than previously recognized. Most patients with this disorder are young, single women who rarely have other compulsive symptoms. Typically, they are extremely embarrassed by their unwanted and senseless behavior. The area from which hair is most often pulled is the scalp, and some victims of this disorder are totally bald. Other areas that may be involved are the eyebrows, eyelashes, and pubic hairs. Sometimes these patients first come to the attention of their primary care physicians or dermatologists, but most persons with trichotillomania can cleverly hide their symptoms and are expert at disguising the effects.

The diagnosis of body dysmorphic disorder (i.e., fear of or overconcern about having a disfigured body) can be even more challenging than that of trichotillomania. The ideas of dysmorphophobic patients may seem delusional. Often, these persons also have other somatoform or psychotic disorders.

In the case of Alvin, it was difficult to determine the correct diagnosis. The compulsive hair pulling and self-view as a grossly disfigured monster would suggest a diagnosis of trichotillomania with dysmorphophobia. The fact that he improved with treatment and that he *welcomed* his improvement supports this diagnosis rather than that of a borderline, somatoform, or other psychotic disorder.

Case Presentation 15
A Conflict With Society

Leon is a 27-year-old, single man who presents with complaints of persistent sexual thoughts of masturbating in public and unwanted ritualized behaviors, including repeated checking of the windows and doors in his house. His checking rituals often prevent him from getting to places on time and are very anxiety-provoking for him if not carried out. Leon was referred to our OCD clinic by his attending psychiatrist for further evaluation and treatment of these complaints.

Leon has been seeing his psychiatrist for approximately 10 years. During that period he was in psychotherapy and was given a number of pharmacotherapeutic agents. At the time of the present evaluation, Leon is being treated with injections of a progestational agent to control his sexual urges to exhibit his genitals and masturbate in public. The progestational agent appears to be helpful in controlling his exhibitionist behavior; however, his urges to masturbate have not diminished. It is noted that Leon's urge to masturbate in public is not a totally ego-dystonic thought and that, by history, the patient reports the act to be quite soothing for him, especially when he is anxious. As previously noted, Leon's checking rituals consist primarily of repeatedly verifying that the doors and windows of his house are locked. He reports that his sleep is disturbed on a nightly basis by obsessive thoughts that some harm will come to him. These thoughts are temporarily neutralized only by the action of checking all door and window locks. This checking ritual is repeated numerous times whenever he leaves the house, and frequently he feels forced to return home several times during the day to recheck the locks.

At the time of the evaluation, the patient also reports having made several suicide attempts, which he claims were secondary to his overall frustration with his compulsions, namely, his checking behaviors, and to the societal constraints that prohibited him from masturbating in public. Leon appears to be slightly dysphoric, and he reports feeling depressed; however, he has no signs or symptoms consistent with a diagnosis of depressive disorder. A comprehensive evaluation suggests no other psychiatric illnesses.

DSM-IV Diagnoses

Axis I: 300.3   Obsessive-Compulsive Disorder
            302.4   Exhibitionism, Moderate

Discussion

At the time of examination, it appeared that Leon suffered from OCD characterized by ritualized checking behavior. This diagnosis was based on the patient's history and high scores on the Yale-Brown Obsessive Compulsive Scale.[1] The Hamilton Depression[2] and Anxiety[3] Rating Scales were also administered. With the additional information provided by these scales, it was determined that Leon did not have depressive symptoms of measurable severity.

[1]Goodman WK, Price LH, Rasmussen SA, et al.: "The Yale-Brown Obsessive Compulsive Scale, I.: Development, Use, and Reliability." *Archives of General Psychiatry* 46:1006–1011, 1989; Goodman WK, Price LH, Rasmussen SA, et al.: "The Yale-Brown Obsessive Compulsive Scale, II.: Validity." *Archives of General Psychiatry* 46:1012–1016, 1989.

[2]Hamilton M: "A Rating Scale for Depression." *Journal of Neurology, Neurosurgery and Psychiatry* 23:56–66, 1960.

[3]Hamilton M: "The Assessment of Anxiety States by Rating." *British Journal of Medical Psychology* 32:50–55, 1959.

The diagnosis of exhibitionism was made based on Leon's 6-month history of recurrent and intense desires to expose his genitals in public and on the fact that he had acted on this desire in the past and found it to be sexually gratifying. Although Leon appears to be distressed by his sexual thoughts, they are not totally ego-dystonic. For this reason, they were determined not to be a manifestation of his OCD.

Case Presentation 16
A Potpourri of Problems

Sara is a 34-year-old, single woman who presents with complaints of obsessive-compulsive symptoms, which first became manifest at age 10 and which have been accompanied by intermittent periods of "incapacitating" anxiety since her early 20s and "mood swings" since her mid-20s. Sara describes unwanted thoughts, including anxiety about having sex with persons in her family, fears that persons around her might become ill, and superstitious thoughts that looking into mirrors might cause bad luck. She also describes ritualized behavior that includes up to 12 hours of house cleaning, repeated hand washing, a need to place perfume in certain areas of the house to counter her concern about filth and dirt, a need to wear certain colors on certain days of the week to avoid bad luck, and overall perfectionism in her house cleaning. Sara states that if she does not perform these rituals, she experiences an incredible amount of anxiety that often incapacitates her. However, she also describes periods of spontaneous anxiety about driving alone and "being stuck" in long lines at the supermarket that are characterized by a racing heart, shortness of breath, fear of going crazy, fear of dying, dizziness, and sweating. On several occasions she says she has "actually passed out." In addition, she gives a history of "mood swings" characterized by depressive symptoms of dysphoria, anhedonia, extreme feelings of hopelessness, suicidal thoughts, hypersomnia, hyperphagia, and periods of decreased energy that last 4 to

6 months at a time. Finally, she describes mood states characterized by extreme irritability, racing thoughts, poor judgment (e.g., she had gone after her father with a butcher knife after a minor criticism), and a decreased need for sleep. At the time of evaluation, Sara reports symptoms of dysphoria, anhedonia, hopelessness, increased appetite, increased sleep, decreased energy, and passive suicidal ideation. Sara's medical history includes diagnoses of thalassemia minor and asthma, but she is not receiving any treatment for these conditions at the time of evaluation.

DSM-IV Diagnoses

Axis I: 300.3   Obsessive-Compulsive Disorder
         296.5x Bipolar I Disorder, Most Recent
                 Episode Depressed
         300.21 Panic Disorder With Agoraphobia

Discussion

On initial evaluation, the patient was given a battery of tests, which included the Yale-Brown Obsessive Compulsive Scale, the Maudsley Obsessional Compulsive Inventory,[4] and the Hamilton Depression and Anxiety Rating Scales. Through a clinical evaluation, which included history taking and a mental status examination, Sara's condition was diagnosed as OCD and, independently, panic disorder with agoraphobic features. Sara claimed that she would spend many hours a day cleaning her house. For that reason, she described herself as being housebound; however, further assessment revealed that she actually became housebound after the onset of the panic attacks and felt more compelled to carry out her cleaning rituals since she now had very little contact with the outside world. Such a relationship between OCD and another anxiety disorder is not uncommon. Comorbidity data from recent studies demonstrate that 15% to 39% of patients with OCD may have experienced panic attacks at some

---

[4]Hodgson RJ, Rachman S: "Obsessional Compulsive Complaints." *Behaviour Research and Therapy* 15:389–395, 1977.

point in their lives, and that panic disorder and agoraphobia develop in some patients with panic attacks. In Sara's case it was also evident that independent of both the panic disorder and the OCD, she had a history consistent with a diagnosis of bipolar disorder and that, at the present time, she appeared to be suffering from depressive disorder.

Case Presentation 17
The Anxious Perfectionist

Ramona is a 24-year-old, single woman who presents with complaints of having intrusive, unwanted thoughts, ritualized checking behavior, problems with perfectionism and procrastination that have interfered significantly with her life and prevented her from pursuing both career and educational goals, and symptoms of "spontaneous anxiety attacks." On initial evaluation, Ramona complains of ego-dystonic thoughts that consist of excessive worry about dirt and germs as well as fear of contracting acquired immunodeficiency syndrome (AIDS). She also has had ego-dystonic sexual thoughts with homosexual content. The homosexual thoughts cause her a great deal of anxiety characterized by restlessness and somatic gastrointestinal symptoms. Ramona claims that the onset of these thoughts occurred approximately 5 years ago. Checking behaviors started during her grade school years; these included checking doors and windows as well as rereading assignments in school to the point that she was evaluated for a learning disability. Although the results of this evaluation were essentially unremarkable, Ramona states that her childhood behaviors had put great pressure on her and had given her feelings of being quite "different." Toward the end of her grade school years, she found herself to be so perfectionistic that she was unable to complete assignments or tasks. At times throughout her high school and college years, she became so preoccupied with single tasks or assignments that there was no possibility of her participating in activities with friends or family. She also developed, in her teen years, a clear inability to make decisions for fear that she would be wrong.

Over the past several years, Ramona has exhibited hoarding behaviors, which consist of collecting old, useless items—even those with no sentimental value. Any attempt at throwing these things away makes her anxious. Finally, at the time of evaluation, Ramona reports symptoms of spontaneous anxiety episodes that occur once or twice a week. These episodes are not accompanied by avoidance behaviors. The episodes, which began in her early 20s, are characterized by palpitations, sweating, extreme nausea, an overwhelming sense of fear, tremulousness, and dizziness. Typically these anxiety attacks last anywhere from 30 to 60 minutes and then gradually subside. Ramona reports no other significant medical or psychiatric history.

DSM-IV Diagnoses

Axis I: 300.3   Obsessive-Compulsive Disorder
            300.01   Panic Disorder Without Agoraphobia
Axis II: 301.4   Obsessive-Compulsive Personality Disorder

Discussion

Ramona presented with clear and obvious symptoms of OCD manifesting as checking behaviors that began during grade school and persisted to the present. In her early 20s she was also preoccupied with obsessional thoughts. In addition, she gave a very clear history of panic attacks that began in her 20s and seemed unrelated to the symptomatology of OCD. The diagnoses of OCD and panic disorder were made on the basis of patient history, the Structured Clinical Interview for DSM-III-R (SCID),[5] and scores on the Yale-Brown Obsessive Compulsive Scale and the Maudsley Obsessional Compulsive Inventory.

[5]Spitzer RL, Williams JBW, Gibbon M, et al.: "The Structured Clinical Interview for DSM-III-R (SCID), I.: History, Rationale, and Description." *Archives of General Psychiatry* 49:624–629, 1992.

Of note are the patient's pathological character symptoms that seem to go hand-in-hand with the OCD symptoms. These include symptoms and complaints of perfectionism, preoccupation with detail, excessive devotion to specific tasks or assignments, and indecisiveness about minor and major decisions, all of which have seriously impeded the occupational, academic, and personal development of the patient. In light of these symptoms, Ramona was also given a diagnosis of obsessive-compulsive personality disorder (OCPD). In the traditional psychoanalytic view of OCD held by many in the past, OCPD was regarded as a predisposing feature of OCD, with the two conditions existing along a continuum. However, this is no longer considered to be the case. In a recent study,[6] OCPD was diagnosed in only 6% of patients with OCD, indicating that OCPD is not invariably a premorbid condition for OCD. In Ramona's case there was an overlapping in the symptomatology of these two conditions. One symptom that could be considered a manifestation of either OCPD or OCD was Ramona's inability to throw out personal possessions. According to DSM-IV criteria, the inability to discard personal possessions is one of the symptoms of OCPD. However, in Ramona's case, the retention of personal possessions was experienced as very ego-dystonic behavior and caused great anxiety. For this reason, her hoarding was considered to be a symptom of OCD rather than of the personality disorder.

Case Presentation 18
Mark's Story

Mark is a 26-year-old, single man who presents with a 17-year history of ritualized counting, touching, hand washing, and tapping accompanied by periodic involuntary grunting, coughing, shoulder

[6]Baer L, Jenike MA, Ricciardi JN, et al.: "Standardized Assessment of Personality Disorders in Obsessive-Compulsive Disorder. *Archives of General Psychiatry* 47:826–830, 1990.

tics, and twitching of the eyes. The patient also states that he has been described as having been a hyperactive child but never received any formal treatment for this complaint. All of these symptoms had waxed and waned during most of Mark's adolescent and adult life but appeared to worsen when he was under any particular stress. As his symptoms worsen, Mark states, he suffers extreme anxiety characterized by sweating, lightheadedness, restlessness, nausea, flushing, and hypervigilance. The onset of these anxiety symptoms is always preceded by an increased stress level or a worsening of motor, vocal, or checking behaviors. Mark's mental status examination at the time of initial evaluation reveals what appears to be involuntary eye twitching and shoulder shrugging. Mark appears to be quite anxious and restless; he verbalizes excessive worry and concern about many areas of his life, including his living situation, his job, and his past relationship with a girlfriend. Although these concerns appear to be legitimate, Mark seems to manifest more psychic and somatic anxiety than would be expected. The patient gives a history of involuntary coughing and grunting with onset at age 9, but these symptoms dissipated during adolescence and had not returned.

DSM-IV Diagnoses

Axis I: 300.3   Obsessive-Compulsive Disorder
            307.23   Tourette's Disorder

Discussion

Mark's initial evaluation consisted of a complete history and physical examination as well as a formal mental status examination. An assessment of his condition was also made based on the results of the Yale-Brown Obsessive Compulsive Scale, the Maudsley Obsessional Compulsive Inventory, and the Hamilton Anxiety and Depression Rating Scales. From this evaluation it was determined that the patient met the criteria for OCD. This determination was based on his symptoms of counting, touching, washing, and tapping, which began early in childhood and followed a waxing and waning pattern throughout his life. The diagnosis of Tourette's disorder was also made, based on the patient's history of having, as a child, exhibited multiple motor and vocal tics. The onset of these symptoms at age 9 and the persistence of the motor tics into adulthood confirmed this diagnosis. Clinicians have long been aware of the overlap between OCD and certain neurological disorders like Tourette's disorder. In fact, Tourette's disorder is associated with obsessive-compulsive symptoms in at least 30% to 40% of patients.[7] Conversely, there have been reports of tic disorder occurring in a (disproportionately) large number of persons with OCD. There was a question of whether or not Mark suffered from concomitant generalized anxiety disorder. However, this diagnosis was not given at the time of evaluation because it was evident from the history and the clinician's observations that the anxiety Mark suffered correlated with an increase in life stressors and/or with worsening of his OCD and/or Tourette's disorder symptoms.

[7]Leckman JF, Walker DE, Goodman WK, et al.: "'Just Right' Perceptions Associated With Compulsive Behavior in Tourette's Syndrome." *American Journal of Psychiatry* 151:675–680, 1994.

CME Test
Chapter 3
Case Presentations 13–18

Please read the six sets of questions (12 questions total) that follow and circle the one best answer for each question on the corresponding answer sheet in the accompanying booklet.

Case Presentation 13: A Counting Nightmare

13A. Compulsions associated with counting are one of the most common symptoms of obsessive-compulsive disorder (OCD). What aspect of this case is somewhat unusual?

1. The patient was extremely intelligent.
2. The patient was able to simultaneously count and engage in conversation.
3. The patient's daughter was the only person who knew about the counting compulsion.

13B. How did this patient manage to minimize the ego-dystonic aspect of her counting compulsion?

1. She kept the disorder a secret from almost everyone around her.
2. She entered her occupational field of choice, though at a lower level than she had originally planned.
3. She derived some satisfaction from demonstrating her counting prowess.

Case Presentation 14: A Diagnostic Dilemma

14A. One differential diagnosis to consider in this case is OCD. What factor rules out this diagnosis?

1. The patient made no attempt to conceal his compulsion to pull out his hair; in fact, he called attention to it.
2. The patient improved in group therapy.

3. The motivation for the hair pulling did not appear to be the prevention of some other anxiety-provoking situation.

14B. What element of this case most strongly suggests that trichotillomania was not the only diagnosis?

1. The patient was preoccupied with the idea that "everybody knows [about] and stares" at his missing eyebrows and eyelashes.
2. The patient was angry with the clinician and his group for not pointing out his condition.
3. The patient's only social contacts were with his mother and his children.

Case Presentation 15: A Conflict With Society

15A. This patient had obsessive sexual thoughts. Why were they not considered a manifestation of his OCD?

1. Sexual pathologies are not usually linked to OCD.
2. The urge to masturbate in public was not totally ego-dystonic for him.
3. The sexual behavior was not ritualized.

15B. What is one DSM-IV criterion for the diagnosis of exhibitionism in this case?

1. Recurrent, intense sexual urges involving touching a nonconsenting person.
2. Recurrent, intense sexual urges involving self-exposure to an unsuspecting stranger.
3. Recurrent, intense sexual urges involving one's own suffering or humiliation.

Case Presentation 16: A Potpourri of Problems

16A. What percentage of patients with OCD have experienced panic attacks at some point in their lives?

1. 10% to 14%
2. 15% to 39%
3. 40% to 70%

16B. Why was the diagnosis of bipolar disorder rather than cyclothymic disorder made in this case?

   1. In cyclothymic disorder, the criteria for major depressive episode are not met.
   2. In bipolar disorder, the patient must have had a hospitalization for manic symptoms.
   3. In cyclothymic disorder, it must be established that the disorder is not related to an organic factor or intoxicating drugs.

Case Presentation 17: The Anxious Perfectionist

17A. What factor in this case suggested that the patient's hoarding behavior was a symptom of OCD rather than of obsessive-compulsive personality disorder?

   1. The comorbidity of panic disorder with the OCD.
   2. The coexistence of checking behaviors.
   3. The ego-dystonic response of the patient to her hoarding.

17B. What aspect of the panic disorder in this case is unusual?

   1. The frequent occurrence of panic attacks (once or twice weekly).
   2. The fact that the panic disorder was not accompanied by agoraphobia.
   3. The fact that the patient was in her early 20s when the panic attacks began.

Case Presentation 18: Mark's Story

18A. What symptoms were the basis for the diagnosis of OCD in this case?

   1. Grunting, coughing, and shoulder twitching.
   2. Counting, touching, hand washing, and tapping.
   3. Sweating, lightheadedness, restlessness, and hypervigilance.

18B. The diagnosis of Tourette's disorder was confirmed by what factor in this case?

   1. The worsening of symptoms in the face of increased life stressors.

2. The fact that comorbidity and overlap of OCD and tic disorders are common.
3. The history of multiple motor and vocal tics in childhood and the persistence of the motor tics in adulthood.

Case Presentation 19
Like Mother, Like Daughter

Anita is an 8-year-old third-grader referred by her family doctor for evaluation and treatment of excessive washing behaviors. Two months before the appointment, Anita's parents noticed that she was washing her hands repeatedly and asking for reassurance about germs. In particular, Anita was concerned that she might have touched her vagina and was extremely worried that she could then touch someone else, spreading some kind of sexual germs. Anita was also very concerned that her bed sheets might be contaminated, and insisted that they be washed at least every other day. Anita's washing behavior had become so frequent that her hands were chapped and cracked from the effects of soap. In addition, she acquired a rather peculiar posture in which she walked and sat with her hands and arms held at chest level for fear that if they were lower she would accidentally touch her vaginal area.

Anita was extremely embarrassed by her obsessions and, at first, refused to discuss them. However, during a play session, the therapist told Anita that they were going to have a "very private talk" on a play telephone. During the conversation the therapist asked her whether she had any strange worries. Anita was then able to describe very briefly her fear of germs. Because of the child's embarrassment, five play sessions were needed to obtain a full description of Anita's obsessions and compulsions.

Despite the seriousness of the symptoms Anita displayed at home, neither her teacher nor her classmates were aware that she had psychiatric problems. Anita's teacher was contacted by the treatment team, and she reported that Anita was very well liked and highly regarded by both students and teachers. She did remark that Anita seemed unusually conscientious and that at times she was prone to worry.

When Anita's parents were asked about any family history of obsessive-compulsive disorder (OCD), her mother admitted that she often felt the need to engage in excessive checking behaviors. She described checking the stove literally hundreds of times to be sure it was off and checking her curling iron in a similar fashion. Anita's mother also described unusual cleaning behaviors, for example, having to get up at 2:00 A.M. to sweep the kitchen floor because of concern that it might have become dirty during the night. Anita's mother had never been treated for OCD, although she admitted the symptoms were upsetting because they consumed so much time. Before the parental intake appointment, she had no idea why she had such unusual "habits."

Only later in treatment did it come to light that Anita's mother also had obsessive thoughts that Anita might have been sexually abused. She would react to these obsessive thoughts by repeatedly interrogating Anita about the possibility of sexual abuse. During these interrogations, Anita's mother would ask questions such as "Are you sure someone has not touched you between your legs?" "Do you think someone might have molested you and you forgot?" "Could someone have touched you in your sleep?" "Your Dad hasn't done something to you, has he?" These interrogations would heighten Anita's anxiety about the "contamination" and lead to further washing behaviors and concern that she was somehow sexually contaminated. Anita's fear of contamination from her vagina seemed to heighten her mother's worry about sexual abuse, and her mother's worry about possible sexual abuse exacerbated Anita's contamination obsessions. This vicious cycle clearly aggravated both the mother's and the daughter's OCD.

DSM-IV Diagnosis

Axis I: 300.3   Obsessive-Compulsive Disorder

Discussion

Most investigators report that 20% to 30% of their patients with
OCD also have a close relative with this condition. Anita's case is
remarkable in that she and her mother have interactive obsessive-
compulsive symptoms that seem to exacerbate the disorder for both
of them. During the year preceding Anita's diagnosis, her mother
had twice taken Anita to a clinic for evaluation of suspected sexual
abuse. In neither instance was there evidence of sexual abuse, but
OCD was not considered. Had a diagnosis of OCD been suspected,
Anita might have received treatment much earlier in the course of
her illness.

Case Presentation 20
Mentally Ill

Rebecca, a 23-year-old, single mother of two, has been brought by
ambulance to the emergency room. An hour earlier, she had reportedly taken an overdose of antidepressants and immediately called
the ambulance for transport to the hospital. Surprisingly, she seems
alert and oriented, with no external signs of distress, and her vital
signs are normal. Rebecca says she took the overdose because she
was angry that no one is doing anything to help her. She states that
although she can live with the knowledge that she is "mentally ill,"
she has asked many times to have plastic surgery so she doesn't
"look" mentally ill, but no one is willing to help her have the surgery.

Further inquiry and review of Rebecca's records indicate that
she has had a long-standing battle with multiple obsessions and
compulsions. She is tormented by constant anxiety-provoking
doubts and obsessions, typically aggressive, that often lead to extended checking rituals. While driving, she frequently has to retrace
her route for many hours to check whether she might have run over
someone, a thought triggered by a vague recollection of going over
a bump on the road. She feels that she cannot trust her own senses

and that her memory is unreliable. The discovery one morning that the latch on her door was open although she was quite certain that she had locked the door the night before led her to conclude that she must have gone out at night and killed someone, a thought that haunted her for over a year.

Rebecca's obsessions that she may have harmed someone have often led her to call the police and inquire about relevant crimes, sometimes insisting that she be arrested as the perpetrator. She is also well known to most mental health agencies in town because she frequently calls them and demands that the severity of her mental illness be recognized and that she be put away in an institution. Often in the past when she has felt ignored or blocked, she has threatened suicide and superficially slashed her wrists in an apparent attempt to force the authorities to take her seriously.

Rebecca has had a troubled and unstable personal life. Her one brief marriage ended in separation and divorce, and she later became pregnant by her ex-husband after a brief postdivorce encounter. She has had other short-term relationships with men, one resulting in her second child. She has never worked and has raised her two children with support from social agencies. Her relationship with her family of origin has been problematic, her feelings toward them alternating between rage and dependence. She has experienced long periods of depressed mood, marked by feelings of emptiness and pervasive uncertainty about her own identity, her feelings, and her life goals.

DSM-IV Diagnoses

Axis I: 300.3   Obsessive-Compulsive Disorder
Axis II: 301.83   Borderline Personality Disorder

Discussion

Rebecca clearly suffers from OCD marked by a long history of malignant obsessive doubts and checking rituals. In addition, her pattern of unstable interpersonal relationships, recurrent suicidal threats (especially in response to perceived abandonment), uncertainty about her identity and goals, and feelings of emptiness justify a diagnosis of borderline personality disorder. Her repeated requests for plastic surgery may also warrant a diagnosis of body dysmorphic disorder, or they may be treated as an aspect of the identity uncertainty of the borderline personality.

Borderline personality disorder is quite atypical in patients with OCD (about 5% in most recent series) but may have prognostic significance. The most commonly diagnosed personality disorders in OCD are from Cluster C (avoidant, dependent, obsessive-compulsive, and passive-aggressive). One recent study,[1] however, has indicated that personality disorders from Clusters A (specifically paranoid and schizotypal) and B (specifically borderline) may be predictors of a negative outcome with behavior therapy and selective serotonin reuptake inhibitors.

Case Presentation 21
Concerns About Safety

Michael is a 55-year-old married man with a long history of multiple fears, which have flared up recently. He also reports feelings of depression and anger, low self-esteem, and suicidal ideation.

Michael is frustrated by his inability to drive his new sports car beyond his neighborhood. The mere thought of driving alone on the highway terrifies him. He fears he might have a panic attack and lose control of the car. He is able to ride in other people's cars with some trepidation and can drive his own car on the highway if a trusted friend or relative is present. Also, Michael cannot spend a night away from home, feeling that he must be home in bed by

---

[1] Baer L, Jenike MA, Black DW, et al.: "Effect of Axis II Diagnoses on Treatment Outcome With Clomipramine in 55 Patients With Obsessive-Compulsive Disorder." *Archives of General Psychiatry* 49:862–866, 1992.

11:30 P.M. to ensure adequate sleep. He does not use public transportation and avoids riding in elevators for fear of being unable to leave if a panic attack should occur. When questioned about these feelings, he denies having actually experienced panic attacks in the past several months.

Michael also reports excessive concern about safety, which leads to extensive checking routines. It takes 20 minutes for him to leave his car in the driveway, because he has to put the transmission into "park" and set the hand brake over and over again to protect against the risk of the car sliding back into the street and hitting someone. He spends several hours every night checking all the windows and doors of his house to prevent burglary and making sure "everything is in place." Michael describes daily incidents of "getting stuck" in front of the door, unable to convince himself that it is securely locked, and manipulating the lock for many minutes until it finally "feels right." Before going to bed, he feels compelled to check his sleeping son to be sure that he is safe. To avoid these malignant worries and rituals, Michael has at times asked his wife to take over the checking routines and then demanded reassurance that they have been done according to his standards.

Michael says his troubles started 30 years ago when he experienced a panic attack while driving on the highway. At the time, he was sure he was having a heart attack. Since this incident, he has had many panic attacks, to which he has responded by avoiding places where panic might catch him unprepared and by developing a variety of rituals. For reasons that are unclear to him, many years ago he began washing his hands 10 to 15 times before going to bed. He also developed an intense fear of not getting enough sleep, which led to his rigid habit of retiring at the same time each night. Michael's extensive checking rituals date back to the same period, and he feels they were motivated by a need to gain control over his life.

Michael describes chronic difficulties in his relationship with his wife, which have brought their marriage to the verge of a breakup. He is unwilling to separate, however, for fear of being left alone.

DSM-IV Diagnoses

Axis I: 300.21   Panic Disorder With Agoraphobia
           300.3   Obsessive-Compulsive Disorder

Discussion

Michael presents a classic history of panic disorder with agoraphobia. Panic attacks, which he initially interpreted as heart attacks, have led to his avoiding situations in which panic may occur with no one available to help him. Michael's agoraphobic avoidance is currently of moderate severity: he is able to leave the house alone, but he is not able to travel for more than a few miles unaccompanied.

Panic disorder with agoraphobia, however, does not account fully for the clinical picture in this case. Michael is preoccupied with concerns about harm, mostly to others, and has adopted a rigid routine of "preventive" checking rituals. These repetitive and time-consuming rituals, which Michael feels compelled to perform, justify a diagnosis of OCD. The tendency to involve family members in rituals and to demand reassurance from them is typical of OCD patients.

The marital difficulties that Michael experiences have contributed to the escalation of his anxiety disorder symptoms (although the reverse may also be true). Typically, in times of great stress, people feel a heightened need to maintain order and control in their lives. In Michael's case, this need translates into an increase in agoraphobic avoidance and compulsive rituals.

Case Presentation 22
The Man With Thoughts
of Sex and Aggression

Eric is a 41-year-old man who has come to the emergency service because he needs a refill of his medication. A review of his record shows that the patient had presented about 18 months earlier with a story of "4 to 5 months of increasing irritability, intrusive thoughts, and loss of interest." The thoughts dealt with homosexuality and with "being mean" and were associated with rituals to ward them off. However, because the patient exhibited "dysphoric mood, loss of interest, loss of energy, self-reproach, and complaints of diminished thinking ability," he was given a diagnosis of major depressive disorder rather than OCD and was given an antidepressant medication.

Eric states that the medication has helped his depression but that he is still far from normal. His chief complaint is that the drug has done nothing to stop his distressing, unwanted, and involuntary thoughts, which are mostly of two types. One pattern of thought is homosexual in content. It is difficult for the patient to give a full description of these thoughts, because often the thoughts are only partially formed. Most of them involve visualizing himself engaging (passively) in a sexual act with a man he admires, of admiring some "masculine" quality in another man, or of being preoccupied with whether he really has had these thoughts. The second type of thought involves women. In contrast to his thoughts with a homosexual pattern, these thoughts are of violent acts toward women, particularly his girlfriend of 10 years. The thoughts might involve actually visualizing something disagreeable happening or the idea that he might be able to visualize such a thing.

Eric describes both thought patterns as occurring more frequently in certain situations, especially when he has just accomplished something. This accomplishment may be a genuine one or merely the passing of a transition point while driving his car, such as a speed limit sign, a bridge, or a town boundary. As a consequence of these thoughts, the patient has developed a tendency to repeat certain of his actions, for example, retracing his route and driving the same boundary over and over again to reassure himself that he could do so without having a bad thought.

Although having described the thought and ritual patterns as being of recent onset, Eric is later able to recall a somewhat similar incident that had taken place some years before. The earlier incident occurred when he was burying a septic tank. He recalled that he had felt compelled to throw the first shovelful of dirt onto the tank and remove it several times because of some discomfort about the fact that he would not be seeing the tank again. This was the only incident of obsessive-compulsive behavior he could recall from the past.

Eric has never married. Although he earned a bachelor's degree in a scientific discipline, he has been in a sales position for 10 years. He says that he does not necessarily want a career in sales but that he does not know what he does want. He denies ever having had homosexual feelings or encounters, although he relates an incident that had occurred 5 years previously in which a male relative had gotten drunk and propositioned him. This experience had shocked him, especially because he had admired the relative and looked upon him as a mentor.

Of interest in his developmental history is that Eric had grown up with another man in the house in addition to his father. Eric describes his father as having been withdrawn and somewhat weak and the other man as having been stronger, more financially successful, and more energetic. After Eric's father died, when the patient was in his 20s, Eric's widowed mother married this other man.

Eric describes himself as fairly likable, friendly, and private, and this is the impression he conveyed during the initial interview. He describes his concentration, sleep, and appetite as normal and notes only a little loss of interest and energy. He is an obese man with an engaging smile, an affable nature, and an appearance of openness. However, it is apparent on longer contact that although he can talk about his symptoms at great length, he has some difficulty talking about his life, particularly the more painful aspects. After months of treatment, for example, when he is asked how things are going, he replies "Fine." It is only after being asked specifically how sales have been that he acknowledges they have been very bad and that he is having trouble paying his bills.

DSM-IV Diagnosis

Axis I: 300.3   Obsessive-Compulsive Disorder

Discussion

The diagnosis of OCD was made on the basis of the patient's chief complaint, which was distressing, intrusive thoughts and the ritualized behaviors that developed as a way of warding off the anxiety these thoughts produced. At the time of this diagnosis, Eric had few signs or symptoms of depression, although the record showed major depressive disorder as his previous diagnosis.

This previous diagnosis indicates the difficulty of differential diagnosis in patients with OCD, who frequently present with dysthymic symptoms. In a patient with such distress over his symptoms, dysphoric mood, self-reproach, and diminished thinking ability would be expected, and yet those symptoms could be interpreted as indications of depression. Had the previous examination included tests for the presence or absence of neurovegetative signs, the test results would have been helpful in the differential diagnosis.

In this case, although the patient demonstrated the isolation of affect of the obsessive-compulsive personality, he did *not* meet most of the criteria for obsessive-compulsive personality disorder or for any other personality disorder, nor did he give the impression on interview of having a personality disorder. This appears to be a case of isolated OCD; nevertheless, psychological antecedents can be hypothesized from the patient's history.

Case Presentation 23
Delusions

Paul, a 60-year-old, is accompanied by his wife and a son, who has arranged the appointment to evaluate his father's obsessive and depressive symptoms. Paul appears depressed and anxious, repeatedly wringing his hands and sighing. He is extremely self-absorbed, responds to direct questions reluctantly, and continually seeks reassurance from family members.

Paul has a long-standing history of OCD, which began at age 8 or 9. His family has indulged him in rituals such as compulsively rechecking the lock on the door, often returning several times from distances as far away as two blocks for that purpose. For years, when the family departed from a motel after staying overnight, Paul would start the engine of the car and then go back to the motel room to check the drawers for possible possessions left behind. According to his wife, he has always been cautious, attentive to details, and rigid, with few, if any, close friends and a limited capacity for warmth and empathy.

Paul's first episode of depression occurred 14 years ago, after he abruptly discontinued fairly heavy alcohol consumption. This episode was tainted with suspicions that his family was maneuvering him into treatment he did not really need and by multiple complaints and demands for attention. He clearly expected to be taken care of and "cured," and when frustrated, he would respond with complaints or angry displays. Paul was successfully treated with electroconvulsive therapy and was able to return to his job at a national company. Over the years, he made successive advancements in that company and was proud of his accomplishments. Five years ago, he opened his own business, and his mood since then was, until a year ago, generally good. According to his family, however, even in the best times he always depended on, and demanded, attention and approval from them.

One year ago, Paul developed severe depression and delusions that his wife was planning to leave him, waitresses were angry with him, and clerks were watching him. Paul repeatedly expressed feelings of inadequacy and insecurity, and he complained about his medications, his physical well-being, and the way he was treated by his family. Despite multiple medications, he has not recovered. Paul still has marked anhedonia; is tearful and shaky, especially in the presence of his family; has lost weight; has decreased energy and interest in all activities; and has apparent concentration and memory dysfunction. He has great difficulty making decisions and states openly that he has lost hope, is worthless, and cannot be helped. He has had thoughts of suicide and at least once has attempted to get out of the car while his wife was driving.

DSM-IV Diagnoses

Axis I: 296.34   Major Depressive Disorder, Recurrent,
                     Severe With Psychotic Features
           300.3   Obsessive-Compulsive Disorder
Axis II: 301.9   Personality Disorder Not Otherwise Specified,
                     With Obsessive-Compulsive and Dependent
                     Features

Discussion

Paul's main presenting symptoms reflect a condition of psychotic depression. His mood is depressed, he has lost interest in all activities, and feels worthless and suicidal. He also feels fatigued and has lost weight, and he has difficulty concentrating. The psychotic character of his depression is shown by the paranoid delusions of being watched or resented by others and betrayed by his family. By history, Paul's condition clearly meets the criteria for OCD, with the patient's having engaged in extensive checking rituals for many years. Without the history, it would have been difficult to make this diagnosis: persons with severe depression often have ruminations that are difficult to distinguish from those of patients with OCD. The comorbidity of depression and OCD is most common; three of four patients with OCD present with some depression at admission, and fully one-third of OCD patients meet the criteria for major depressive disorder.

In addition, Paul's long-standing personality characteristics and interpersonal style, which also manifest themselves in his current illness, justify a diagnosis of a personality disorder. Paul is described as being rigid, interpersonally distant, overly attentive to details, suspicious, insecure, indecisive, and dependent, and as having an extreme need for approval. Therefore, a diagnosis of mixed personality disorder with obsessive-compulsive and dependent features seems most appropriate. These Cluster C personality features are also among the most commonly diagnosed personality disorder features in patients with OCD.

Case Presentation 24
Too Many Zits

Michael, a 13-year-old high school freshman, was referred to a child psychiatrist by his dermatologist, who felt that Michael's concern about his acne was excessive. After careful consideration, the dermatologist had refused to provide further treatment for Michael's acne without psychiatric consultation. Michael agreed that his worries about his face were "excessive," but he disagreed that he needed to see a psychiatrist, stating, "I'm not crazy."

Like many other adolescents, Michael developed mild acne vulgaris at puberty. Although his acne was not objectively severe enough to warrant aggressive treatment with medications, Michael *felt* that his face was severely disfigured by acne, and yet *knew* that his acne was neither worse nor better than that of many of his peers. Michael found that his preoccupation with facial disfigurement, coupled with the fear that he would be unattractive to girls his age, was initially easy to stifle. However, when a female classmate in whom he was interested began to date an older boy, Michael began to experience thoughts about acne that were intensely dysphoric. Driven by his feelings, Michael began a nightly ritual directed to "correcting the problem," including washing his face, applying over-the-counter acne creams, and squeezing his comedones and acne pustules. In reality, Michael knew that these measures made his face look even worse, producing more acne, increased redness, and very dry and chapped skin. Eventually, Michael's mother took him to the dermatologist, who prescribed conventional topical acne treatments. Despite showing objective improvement with medical treatment, Michael demanded a prescription for an oral antiacne medication that several of his friends had taken with good results. Fortunately, Michael's dermatologist recognized the unreasonableness of this request and referred him to a child psychiatrist. By this time, Michael was spending several hours at night and less time in the morning (because his parents made him catch the school bus) performing his acne rituals.

Although quite demoralized by his symptoms, Michael reacted hopefully to the psychiatrist's careful explanation of his condition and improved dramatically with combined drug and behavior therapy.

DSM-IV Diagnosis

Axis I: 300.7   Body Dysmorphic Disorder
                    (Dysmorphophobia)

Discussion

This case illustrates one of the most common obsessive-compulsive spectrum disorders. Michael evidenced a single symptom focused on a postulated physical abnormality rather than the typical obsessions and compulsions found in OCD. Thus, body dysmorphic disorder, one of the somatoform disorders, is the appropriate DSM-IV diagnosis. Nevertheless, the phenomenological similarity between OCD and body dysmorphic disorder, coupled with the fact that this somatoform disorder responds readily to the same treatments used in OCD, argues that body dysmorphic disorder may be a variant of OCD.

Interestingly, body dysmorphic disorder is not infrequently seen in adolescents; in fact, pore and skin picking related to acne vulgaris is the most common presenting complaint of adolescents with a somatoform disorder. Other common obsessions include concerns about the size of particular body parts, such as the nose, buttocks, penis, or breasts. Corollary compulsions include intervening cosmetically and repeatedly inspecting the offending body part and seeking reassurance about its normality. Common comorbid conditions include social phobia, substance abuse, and major depressive disorder.

CME Test
Chapter 4
Case Presentations 19–24

Please read the six sets of questions (12 questions total) that follow and circle the one best answer for each question on the corresponding answer sheet in the accompanying booklet.

Case Presentation 19: Like Mother, Like Daughter

19A. Why is this case of obsessive-compulsive disorder (OCD) unusual?

1. The patient developed OCD symptoms at a young age.
2. The patient and her mother have interactive obsessive-compulsive symptoms.
3. The patient's OCD was completely unsuspected by her teacher or other students.

19B. What percentage of patients with OCD are reported to have close relatives with the condition?

1. 10% to 15%
2. 40% to 50%
3. 20% to 30%

Case Presentation 20: Mentally Ill

20A. Although borderline personality disorder is uncommon in patients with OCD, its comorbid presence with OCD may be significant with respect to what aspect of such a case?

1. Such patients tend to engage in repetitive violent acts and are more likely to require hospitalization.
2. Such patients are less likely to be helped by behavior therapy or selective serotonin reuptake inhibitors.
3. Such patients tend to have troublesome, persistent thoughts of having harmed someone that have no real basis.

20B. Despite the clear comorbidity of OCD and borderline personality disorder, what features of this case presentation underlie the diagnosis of OCD?

1. The obsessions of harming others and the checking rituals.
2. The patient's being divorced.
3. The repeated requests for inpatient treatment.

Case Presentation 21: Concerns About Safety

21A. Many of this patient's concerns involve his car. What aspect of these concerns is specifically related to his OCD?

1. Inability to drive the car on the highway without another person present.
2. The need to repeatedly set the transmission and parking brake when the car is in the driveway.
3. Fear of losing control of the car.

21B. This patient denies having experienced panic attacks in the past several months. Why does this fact not invalidate the diagnosis of panic disorder?

1. The patient also suffers from OCD, a common comorbid condition.
2. The patient's avoidance of traveling alone in the car reflects a fear of panic attacks.
3. The patient's repeated safety checking indicates a fear of panic attacks.

Case Presentation 22: The Man With Thoughts of Sex and Aggression

22A. Many patients with OCD, like this patient, have dysthymic symptoms, yet the diagnosis in this case was isolated OCD. Why was there no secondary diagnosis of major depressive disorder?

1. Most patients with OCD have a dysphoric mood because of their distressing obsessive-compulsive symptoms.

2. The patient's depression was previously helped by antidepressant medication, but his obsessive thoughts persisted.
3. The patient had few signs or symptoms of depression at the time of the diagnosis of OCD.

22B. What was the significance of the homosexual and violent content of this patient's obsessive thoughts to the diagnosis of OCD?

1. The patient was apparently angry at his mother for having remarried after the death of his father.
2. There was no significance to the content of the obsessive thoughts in terms of the diagnosis of OCD.
3. The patient's father had been withdrawn and weak, and therefore the patient felt drawn toward other men who were more "masculine" than his father had been.

Case Presentation 23: Delusions

23A. Ruminations in the context of major depressive disorder may make it difficult to recognize coexisting OCD. What factor helps determine that the two conditions coexist in this case?

1. The patient's obsessive paranoid delusions.
2. The patient's multiple complaints and demands for attention.
3. The patient's long-standing history of obsessive-compulsive checking rituals.

23B. What characteristics in this case justify an Axis II diagnosis of personality disorder not otherwise specified, with obsessive-compulsive and dependent features?

1. The patient's extensive checking rituals of many years' duration.
2. The patient's qualities of maintaining interpersonal distance and indecisiveness.
3. The patient's ruminations about not being cared for by his family.

Case Presentation 24: Too Many Zits

24A. Why was this patient given the diagnosis of body
dysmorphic disorder and not delusional disorder, somatic
type?

1. The patient demanded inappropriately potent medication
for his condition.
2. The slight physical anomaly is perceived by the patient as
severe disfigurement.
3. The patient can acknowledge the possibility that his
concerns about his physical defect are excessive.

24B. What is the phenomenological similarity between OCD and
body dysmorphic disorder referred to in the discussion of
this case?

1. The common occurrence among adolescents of obsessive
concerns about the size of body parts such as the buttocks,
nose, breasts, or penis.
2. The fact that the patient had only a single symptom.
3. The patient's excessive concern with his acne and
indulgence in special rituals to treat it.

Case Presentation 25
The Boy Who Turned Right

Joey, an 8-year-old third-grader, was by all accounts a normal youngster until his maternal grandfather died. Joey had been especially close to this grandfather, who often took him to the park, where the two would spend the afternoon fishing. At first Joey reacted to his grandfather's death with disbelief; then, at his grandfather's funeral, he burst into tears, circling the casket several times (to the right) in a way that appeared as if he were trying somehow to find a vantage point from which to observe his grandfather coming back to life.

For months after the funeral, Joey was not really himself. He didn't seem depressed, and his teachers reported that he played well with the other children. Rather, he seemed preoccupied, although no one knew exactly with what. Eventually, Joey's mother noticed that it took him a long time to make his way around the house. He also became increasingly stubborn, especially when the family was away from home. The reason for Joey's slowness soon became apparent: Joey would turn only to the right. Once, when he wasn't aware that his mother was watching, Joey marched to the right around and around the kitchen table, counting to himself as he turned and finally stopping with a sigh of relief. From this moment on, when his mother attempted to get him to turn with her to the left, tantrums would follow. Finally it was understood that Joey's refusal to turn any way but to the right accounted for his slowness and for most instances of oppositional behavior.

When asked about turning right, Joey initially denied that he was doing things any differently from how he had always done them. Later, however, he confided to his mother that he worried a lot about the possibility that his father might die and that turning right, especially in circles, was one way to prevent this from happening. Although Joey wished he didn't have to turn right to safeguard his father, he insisted that he was being helpful in doing so. Joey made no connection between the death of his grandfather and the development of his worries or his "turning right" ritual.

DSM-IV Diagnosis

Axis I: 300.3   Obsessive-Compulsive Disorder

Discussion

This case nicely illustrates several features that are common to childhood-onset obsessive-compulsive disorder (OCD): 1) a preponderance of males in the younger age range, 2) motoric rituals related to sensory incompleteness, and 3) onset after a stressful event. It also illustrates the lack of insight common in younger children with OCD, although, interestingly, most children, like Joey, remain embarrassed by their symptoms. In contrast to OCD of early onset, OCD beginning in adolescence occurs equally often in males and females, involves washing rituals in response to contamination obsessions in over 80% of patients, and is more likely to have a spontaneous onset.

Early-onset OCD may have a slightly higher familial incidence—in retrospect, Joey's maternal grandmother appears to have been a "washer"—and possibly shares a psychopathological border with Tourette's disorder, chronic motor tic disorder, and perhaps a subtype of attention-deficit/hyperactivity disorder (ADHD). Joey's turning right instead of left may represent a conditioned response (he turned right around the casket). Alternatively, it is quite possible that it represents a subtle form of left-sided neglect, reflecting dysfunction in Joey's right hemisphere. Evidence for the latter includes a higher-than-expected prevalence of left-sided neurological "soft signs" and abnormalities in visuospatial processing in children with OCD.[1] In adults, similar neurological impairments have been associated with greater obsessionality and, perhaps, with resistance to pharmacotherapy. In contrast, these findings in children with OCD have no demonstrated prognostic significance.

Case Presentation 26
Fearing the Menstrual Flow

Laura, a 22-year-old woman, was admitted to a psychiatry unit for evaluation and treatment of cyclically occurring obsessions and compulsions. Two years before admission, the patient developed toxic shock syndrome (TSS). At that time, she informed her physician that she had been wearing tampons every day of the month since menarche because she feared beginning her menses unprepared and staining her underwear with blood. Laura recovered from TSS, and her physician strongly discouraged further tampon use.

After discontinuing daily use of tampons, Laura began to verbalize fears that she would begin her menses unprepared. Her fears were limited to the week preceding the onset of menses and to the menstrual period itself. During this phase of her cycle, Laura continually asked her mother whether she, Laura, had blood on her clothes, what would happen if her sanitary napkin slipped out of place, and whether others were aware she was menstruating. To prepare herself for her menstrual period, Laura would spend nearly 4 hours in the bathroom several times a day performing an elaborate ritual to be sure she had properly applied her sanitary napkin. She would remove the adhesive strip from a sanitary napkin and, after placing it in her underwear, would run her finger down the center

---

[1]March JS, Johnston H, Jefferson JW, et al.: "Do Subtle Neurological Impairments Predict Treatment Resistance to Clomipramine in Children and Adolescents With Obsessive-Compulsive Disorder?" *Journal of Child and Adolescent Psychopharmacology* 1:133–140, 1990.

of the napkin while counting to 7. She would then pinch the anterior end of the napkin while counting to 7 and repeat the same for the posterior end of the napkin. Next, she would tug on each corner of the napkin while counting to 50. Laura repeated this ritual up to 4 hours at a time. During the premenstrual and menstrual phases of her cycle, she appeared depressed and anxious, refused to leave her parents' home, and avoided social contact except when asking for reassurance about her menstrual period. As soon as her menses was over, the obsessional thinking and compulsive rituals ended. She would then revert to her usual personality, becoming outgoing, talkative, and happy; at such times she enjoyed dancing, roller skating, reading, and watching television. In addition, she was able to work as a child care assistant.

During Laura's hospitalization on the psychiatry unit, her premenstrual and menstrual behavior was observed. Unless encouraged to leave her room, the patient spent the entire day lying on her bed crying or in the bathroom checking her underwear for blood. She refused to eat and avoided all social contact. She continually asked for reassurance that she would receive help using sanitary napkins once her menstrual period began. Physicians and nursing staff found it difficult, if not impossible, to redirect Laura from her obsessional thinking to other topics of conversation. She repeated the following phrases whenever she was approached by a staff member, "My mind is totally on how to put the pad on. I completely have no sense of what to do when the time comes. My mind is totally gone. I don't know what to do about the blood." As her parents had described, her affect was anxious and depressed, and she expressed the wish to commit suicide. However, within 1 to 2 days after her menstrual period ended, her behavior changed dramatically. Laura became cheerful and outgoing; she enjoyed ward activities and interacted normally with staff, with patients, and with family members. Interestingly, when she was "back to normal," she had no memory of her behavior during the premenstrual and menstrual phases of her cycle.

Computed tomography and magnetic resonance imaging studies of the patient's head were normal, as were the results of sleep-deprived electroencephalography and lumbar puncture. Laura's complete blood count and chemistry panel were also normal. Hypothyroidism, diagnosed at age 19, was being managed appropriately with levothyroxine. Neuropsychological testing showed borderline low intelligence but no lateralizing findings.

Past medical history was significant for three febrile seizures in childhood and two grand mal seizures in late adolescence. In addition, Laura had severe periodontal disease. Because the patient was adopted, no information about illness in her biological family members was available.

DSM-IV Diagnoses

Axis I: 300.3   Obsessive-Compulsive Disorder
Axis II: V62.89   Borderline Intellectual Functioning
Axis III: Hypothyroidism

Discussion

The patient's symptoms met the criteria for OCD as defined in DSM-IV. Laura experienced recurrent obsessions and compulsions of sufficient severity to cause her marked distress, consume a great deal of time, and significantly interfere with her social and occupational functioning. At the time of hospitalization, the patient did not recognize her behavior as excessive or unreasonable.

Although Laura's condition was diagnosed as OCD, her symptom pattern appeared to differ from that commonly seen in OCD. The intensity of OCD symptoms may wax and wane in many patients, but intermittent symptoms linked to the menstrual cycle and separated by asymptomatic intervals are uncommon. In this instance, not only the timing of the patient's symptoms linked to the menstrual cycle but also the content of her obsessions and compulsions was limited to issues involving menstruation. Although many psychiatric disorders, such as major depressive disorder, may worsen premenstrually, it is unusual for patients to experience symptoms strictly limited to the premenstrual and menstrual phases. (Premenstrual dysphoric disorder is an exception.) This case also differs from many cases of OCD because the patient had no memory of her obsessive-compulsive behavior when she was asymptomatic.

Case Presentation 27
The Family Held Hostage

Dick, a 14-year-old, was brought to the clinic because of his recent threat to commit suicide. Dick's parents were to leave in a few days on a business trip but had found a suicide note, a noose made of clothesline, and several butcher knives in Dick's room. When confronted, Dick told his parents that he simply did not want them to go on this trip and that he really did not intend to kill himself. Dick went on to say that he was extremely afraid that his parents might be killed in a plane crash.

Dick's parents had first noticed he was having problems about 3 years before this incident. At that time, he would repeatedly switch lights on and off, open and close car doors, backtrack after going upstairs, and engage in peculiar movements in which he would touch his chin and chest. Over time, Dick gradually became more and more concerned that some harm might befall his parents. He was increasingly insistent that they not travel, and he would feign a variety of illnesses in an attempt to keep them at home.

Dick presented as an alert, appropriately dressed, tall, thin adolescent who sat quietly during the initial part of the interview with his parents. When questions were directed at him, Dick was able to answer appropriately. His speech was clear, and he expressed his thoughts logically and coherently. There was no evidence of a thought disorder. Dick described his mood as generally happy, and his affect was appropriate. When his parents were excused, Dick was able to talk somewhat more openly about his obsessions and compulsions. He admitted that the thoughts and rituals were "somewhat silly" and that he would like to be rid of them. He also expressed some fear that by coming to see a psychiatrist, he would be viewed as "a psycho."

When his parents returned, Dick again became very tense. His father, a successful, hard-driving businessman, immediately demanded, "What is this nonsense all about?" His mother sat silently with a sad expression on her face. Both parents denied any family history of anxiety disorders; however, Dick's mother had been hospitalized 2 years earlier for suicidal feelings related to depression, and Dick's father was recovering from alcoholism and had been sober for 8 years.

DSM-IV Diagnosis

Axis I: 300.3   Obsessive-Compulsive Disorder

Discussion

This is an unusual presentation of adolescent OCD in that the chief complaint was a suicidal threat. Typically, suicidality is not part of the clinical picture of OCD unless the patient has a concomitant major depressive episode.

Control issues within the family are frequently problematic when one of the family members has OCD. In this case, control issues arose out of the child's attempts to force other family members to forego travel to decrease his obsessional worry about fatal accidents. What initially appeared to be suicidality was found actually to be a struggle for control within the family. This family probably had difficulties with control issues before the onset of the patient's OCD. Although it is unlikely that family dynamics play a causal role in OCD, these issues can be complicating factors. When treating OCD in patients of all ages, the clinician should be sensitive to intrafamily conflicts and struggles, because they may have an important impact on treatment outcome.

Case Presentation 28
The Chemistry Teacher

Lucille was sent to the hospital emergency room by her family clinician to be admitted for psychiatric observation. She was a petite 57-year-old woman who taught high school chemistry. Lucille complained of acute panic symptoms and expressed relief when asked to sign in to the voluntary psychiatric inpatient unit.

Further evaluation revealed that Lucille's husband, age 63, also a school teacher, had had a stroke about 6 months before her admission. He had been in care facilities since the stroke occurred but was now scheduled to return home. Lucille's panic was induced by thoughts of having to change the wet sheets, diapers, and under-wear of her now incontinent husband.

In successive meetings, Lucille also revealed that for years she had had a counting compulsion while she washed. Each area of her body was given a certain number of strokes with the soap, although the greatest number of strokes were applied to the pubic area. Interestingly, she and her husband had had a good love life. She reported no difficulty in dealing with sexual "fluids," only with urine.

With appropriate medication, Lucille was able to leave the hospital after 18 days and to care for her husband when he returned home. Her progress continued during succeeding months, and even-tually she was seen only on a periodic basis.

Three years later Lucille telephoned the hospital again in great anxiety and panic, begging to be admitted. When pressed for a reason, she reported that her daughter had just announced her engagement and was going to marry within the year. Lucille was worried about what would happen if her daughter got pregnant, had the baby, and asked her to baby-sit. The thought of changing the baby's diapers had again produced a panic reaction.

DSM-IV Diagnosis

Axis I: 300.3   Obsessive-Compulsive Disorder

Discussion

This intelligent woman, a teacher of high school chemistry, exhibited both an obsession and a compulsion. The obsession presented itself almost as if it were a phobia. She was preoccupied with the dangers of urine, but what she was actually preoccupied with was *her perception* of the dangers of urine. During several years of therapy, it was impossible to determine what she thought urine could do to harm her. In teaching her chemistry class, she had to handle acids and other more dangerous chemicals on a regular basis and was able to do so without fear. Moreover, she did not seem to be bothered by other body fluids.

Lucille's compulsion had two elements that are very typical: washing and counting. She was compelled to stroke each body part with soap a certain number of times as she washed it. The pubic area required the most attention (i.e., 30 strokes). If time was short, she would rather be late than wash herself inadequately in spite of the fact that punctuality was very much a part of her makeup.

Case Presentation 29
The Redhead

Eleanor, a 38-year-old woman, presented with the complaint that "everything is a chore." She reported that she felt no interest in things, could not concentrate, and had slowed down considerably over the past 2 years. Although she seemed to be physically attractive, she was dressed in thick wool clothing of dull, drab color. However, her hair was dyed red, calling attention to her in a way that contradicted her mode of dress.

Eleanor reported that she was the product of a religiously mixed marriage. Her father, a retired military sergeant, was a prominent Jewish leader, and her mother was an Irish Catholic. She and her three siblings were raised in the Catholic faith. Her father was physically abusive to her mother and her younger sister. However, he favored Eleanor and never hit her or her two younger brothers. Eleanor had faint memories of being sexually abused by her maternal grandmother, who was an alcoholic. She was too frightened ever to tell her mother of this incident. In addition, she thought she was the victim of date rape at age 16, although she seems to have had a dissociative reaction and could give no description of the incident.

Eleanor married at age 19. She described her husband as an accountant of Irish background—very athletic and good looking—and reported their sexual relations to be "very pleasurable." She took great pride in their two fine, well-adjusted children, whom she described as "artistic in nature."

The patient was given medication for depression and was followed in psychotherapy. During the course of the therapeutic sessions, other symptoms began to emerge. She admitted to being extremely perfectionistic, with a need for neatness, cleanliness, and symmetry. She reported the need to keep all the drapes and curtains closed. If the doorbell rang, she would not answer it if the rooms did not measure up to her standards. She also described several symmetry rituals. For example, she reported that she was continually forced to rearrange the items on her dresser so that a photograph of her family would directly face the door and be at precise angles to the ginger jar and lamp. If there was any disturbance in this arrangement, she felt an uneasiness about the well-being of some member of the family.

After several months of therapy, Eleanor also admitted that, on a regular basis, she pulled out her hair, strand by strand, over a period of many hours. The hair pulling was confined to only one area, which was well concealed. She confided that not even her husband had ever realized what she was doing. Again, after several months, she sheepishly made another admission: she ate the follicles of the pulled hairs. There was great guilt surrounding this activity, and she fully expected dire punishment, "here" or "in the hereafter."

DSM-IV Diagnoses

Axis I: 300.3   Obsessive-Compulsive Disorder
           300.4   Dysthymic Disorder
           312.39   Trichotillomania
Axis II: 301.4   Obsessive-Compulsive Personality Disorder

Discussion

The patient presented with symptoms that suggested dysthymic disorder. Indeed, this diagnosis was warranted on the basis of Eleanor's depressed mood of 2 years' duration, low self-esteem, poor concentration, low energy, and feelings of hopelessness. It appeared later that her depression was secondary to obsessive-compulsive symptoms and trichotillomania. The diagnosis of OCD was made on the basis of Eleanor's cleaning and symmetry rituals. The OCD was complicated by obsessive-compulsive personality disorder, which was characterized by a pervasive pattern of perfectionism and an adherence to overly strict and often unattainable standards expressed primarily in compulsive housecleaning. The trichotillomania was apparent from the scalp alopecia resulting from hours of strand-by-strand hair pulling. Interestingly, the patient pulled hair strands only from the right parietal area and carefully hid the affected area from her family. Despite reports that trichotillomania is more common in children than adults, Eleanor did not develop symptoms until her mid-30s. It is also interesting to note that although dysthymic disorder was secondary to trichotillomania and OCD in this patient, the depressive symptoms represented the presenting complaint and were the more obvious. As is frequently the case, Eleanor kept the symptoms of OCD and trichotillomania hidden for as long as possible both from her family and from the clinician.

Case Presentation 30
John's Story

John, a 26-year-old, single man, was referred by another psychiatrist for treatment evaluation. John traced his problems to his first sexual experience 9 years earlier when the girl's mother found the young couple in bed together. At the time, John was confused and anxious and suffered from headaches, but he confided in no one. He later enlisted in the navy but was granted a psychiatric discharge at age 19 or 20. During the next 2½ years he attended college as a classics major until he was forced to drop out because of almost constant and severe depression. Before the present referral, he had been evaluated and treated psychodynamically and had received a variety of antidepressant medications. Highly verbal and introspective, he was obsessed with his own thought processes as well as with sexual fantasies and with violent and bodily images. For years John had been, in a sense, committed to the perpetuation of his illness and resistant to all forms of treatment. During the course of psychotherapy it also became apparent that John had a personality disorder with narcissistic and passive-aggressive features.

The following is a verbatim example of John's thinking, which is readily characterizable as introspective, self-centered, intellectual, and verbally precise:

"There is anxiety; but it is not the root of the malady. Rather it is the strange significance which things—a whole assortment of things and ideas—take on in my fevered perception. Oh, I know better, and am fully aware that my thinking, my cognition, is not as it should be (without quite knowing how it should be, so that while I know what behavior and thinking is 'inappropriate,' I'm far from certain what is appropriate). I am able to pull my mind back from its strange wanderings, but am so frequently obliged to do so that I can never usefully employ it. I am constantly aware of my own stubborn abstraction, and so anxious not to show it while at the same time searching my shredded consciousness for clues as to how I should be behaving and 'seeming' under the various conditions in which I find myself, that I am generally in a state of absolute confusion, self-consciousness, and anxiety.

"When the illness began to make itself apparent to me (at which time I fully believed that I was either going mad or becoming the most abandoned sort of pervert) it was not connected with any overt anxiety. I mean that although it made me anxious, it did not have an anxiety component independent of my reflections on it. The development of a sort of independent anxiety problem came later."

DSM-IV Diagnoses

Axis I:	300.3	Obsessive-Compulsive Disorder
	296.3x	Major Depressive Disorder, Recurrent
Axis II:	301.9	Personality Disorder Not Otherwise Specified, With Narcissistic and Passive-Aggressive Features

Discussion

The diagnosis was made after the patient's hospitalization on the basis of his observed behavior, history, and verbalizations. John's OCD took the form of obsessive thoughts. He would spend hours thinking, speaking, and writing about his condition and mental processes. As is typical of the patient with OCD, John's mental view was ego-dystonic. As he expressed it at one point, "I wish I would become psychotic so I wouldn't know I'm crazy." This has also been described as the "feel right" phenomenon in which the patient is aware that the quality of thinking doesn't "feel right."

Over a period of time, the patient has remained dysfunctional, and although he has constantly asked for help and expressed willingness to try anything, he remains doubtful that anything will really help, and frightened as much by the thought that he might get well as by the idea of remaining ill.

CME Test
Chapter 5
Case Presentations 25–30

Please read the six sets of questions (12 questions total) that follow and circle the one best answer for each question on the corresponding answer sheet in the accompanying booklet.

Case Presentation 25: The Boy Who Turned Right

25A. What criterion for obsessive-compulsive disorder (OCD), usually met in adult patients, is "waived" in this case because the patient is a child?

  1. The person recognizes that his behavior is excessive or unreasonable.
  2. The behavior is designed to neutralize or prevent discomfort or a dreaded event but is not connected in a realistic way to the event.
  3. The behavior is performed according to certain rules.

25B. How was this case different from OCD cases with onset in adolescence?

  1. Many more males than females experience the onset of OCD in adolescence.
  2. Washing rituals are part of the symptomatology in most adolescent patients with OCD.
  3. A stressful event usually triggers the onset of OCD in adolescents.

Case Presentation 26: Fearing the Menstrual Flow

26A. This patient's symptoms failed to meet the DSM-IV criteria for obsessions because she apparently did not perceive her obsessions as intrusive and senseless, nor did she attempt to repress them. Why is the diagnosis of OCD nevertheless valid in this case?

  1. The DSM-IV criteria for OCD do not require that the patient perceive the obsessions as intrusive.

2. The case fulfills the DSM-IV criteria for compulsions.
3. The patient refused social contact during her premenstrual and menstrual phase.

26B. What is the most unusual aspect of this OCD case?

1. The concomitant diagnoses of borderline intellectual functioning and hypothyroidism.
2. The patient's anxious and depressed affect while she was symptomatic.
3. The cyclic nature of the symptoms and the patient's amnesia for them.

Case Presentation 27: The Family Held Hostage

27A. What factor in this case suggested a diagnosis of OCD rather than major depressive disorder?

1. The patient's fear of being seen as a "psycho."
2. The fact that the patient expressed himself logically and coherently.
3. The patient's history of rituals connected with fear of his parents' traveling.

27B. This patient's reason for presenting was a suicide threat. What is a possible explanation for this behavior in the absence of a diagnosis of depression?

1. The rope and knives were part of the patient's compulsive rituals.
2. The suicide threat reflected a control struggle within the patient's family.
3. Suicidality is a common presenting feature of adolescent OCD.

Case Presentation 28: The Chemistry Teacher

28A. Specific phobia was not considered as a diagnosis in this case. What possible element of the history justifies this diagnostic decision?

1. The patient had washing and counting compulsions.

2. The patient had no difficulty dealing with body fluids other than urine.
3. The patient was stabilized with appropriate medication and was able to care for her incontinent husband on his return home.

28B. This case is typical of OCD in what way?

1. The rituals of washing and counting.
2. The patient's obsession despite being an intelligent person.
3. The patient's fear of a body fluid.

Case Presentation 29: The Redhead

29A. What was the basis of the dual diagnosis of OCD and obsessive-compulsive personality disorder in this case?

1. The patient had symmetry rituals and obsessions about house cleaning, as well as a pervasive pattern of perfectionism.
2. The patient failed to inform her family or the therapist about her compulsive symptoms for as long as possible.
3. Secondary dysthymic disorder was present.

29B. What was the basis of the Axis I diagnosis of dysthymic disorder?

1. The patient's tendency to keep her trichotillomania secret from family members and her clinician.
2. The patient's low self-esteem, poor concentration, low energy, and feelings of hopelessness.
3. The patient's guilt about her consumption of her hair follicles.

Case Presentation 30: John's Story

30A. This case is different from most cases of OCD, and the diagnosis is perhaps somewhat more difficult, because of the focus of the patient's obsessions. What was that focus?

1. His failure in the navy and subsequent psychiatric discharge.

2. Fear of being caught again, as he was during his first sexual experience.
3. The content and self-analysis of his own thoughts.

30B. Why does the prognosis appear to be poor for this patient?

1. He suffers from multiple illnesses (OCD, recurrent major depression, and personality disorder not otherwise specified, with narcissistic and passive-aggressive features) that have responded poorly to previous treatment.
2. His OCD symptoms have been present for many years.
3. The onset of his OCD was associated with a precipitating event.

Case Presentation 31
Compulsive Cutting

Sherry, a 16-year-old, was referred for outpatient treatment by her school guidance counselor because of refusal to go to school. Since age 8, Sherry has had typical obsessive-compulsive disorder (OCD) symptoms, including fear of germs and hand-washing rituals. By age 15 she was washing her hands 4 to 5 hours per day. Her symptoms came to clinical attention when she refused to attend school because she could not use the school bathroom.

Like most patients whose OCD is newly diagnosed, Sherry was relieved to learn about OCD. She complied readily with treatment, and her contamination obsessions and washing rituals responded well to a combination of pharmacotherapy and exposure and re-sponse prevention. Three months after entering treatment, she was able to return to school full time.

Six months later, pharmacotherapy was discontinued and booster behavior therapy was initiated. Sherry continued to do well for several months but then called frantically to report the develop-ment of a compulsive urge to cut herself. Interviews with Sherry and her parents uncovered no evidence of emotional, physical, or sexual abuse.

When closely questioned about this new symptom, Sherry reported an obsession ("Cut yourself"), a corresponding urge to act on the obsession, and intensely dysphoric affects involving a mixture of fear and anger. With the development of the urge to self-mutilate came a variety of avoidance behaviors. First she began to avoid knives and then scissors and razors, and then she quickly became unable to go into the kitchen. Sherry had no history of prior aggressive obsessions; she was frightened and confused by these new symptoms. Nevertheless, although she had lightly scratched herself on one occasion for symptom relief, she was generally able to resist the urge to harm herself. In this context, she found the entire experience to be intensely ego-dystonic. Sherry did not meet the criteria for any DSM-IV Axis I disorder other than OCD, and she denied suicidality or homicidality.

Sherry was again treated with pharmacotherapy and with exposure and response prevention. The latter consisted of preventing avoidance rituals, first with therapist-assisted and then with patient-directed exposure to knives, scissors, and razors. She responded well to these interventions and remains in remission with pharmacotherapy, which she wishes to continue.

DSM-IV Diagnosis

Axis I: 300.3   Obsessive-Compulsive Disorder

Discussion

Aggressive urges toward others are not uncommon in patients with OCD; aggressive obsessions toward the self are less common but not rare. These terrifying symptoms present a difficult diagnostic picture for the treating mental health professional. The probability of a history of previous physical or sexual abuse and related Axis II psychopathology is high in patients who self-mutilate. It is also high in patients with a depressive-spectrum illness. However, in these patients, the urge to self-mutilate almost always serves to communicate a complex mixture of revenge and dependency needs. Even in the presence of this picture, the clinician should consider OCD in differential diagnosis, because OCD can occur in the context of a trauma-related or depressive-spectrum illness. In addition, even when a case of OCD is complicated by comorbidity with an Axis I or Axis II disorder, or both, the combination of standard behavioral and pharmacotherapeutic interventions is usually effective treatment for the OCD.

Case Presentation 32
Shopping for the Number 4

Sally, a 22-year-old college student, presented with self-described "trouble shopping." She simply could not make up her mind what or how much to buy and so left shopping to her roommates. When forced to shop, she relied on a ritual involving the number 4, sometimes buying in 4s, other times avoiding buying anything connected with 4 or multiples of 4. Initially treated with insight-oriented psychotherapy without benefit, she sought treatment for OCD after reading *The Boy Who Couldn't Stop Washing*, by Judith L. Rapoport, M.D.

On careful questioning, Sally reported that OCD symptoms had been present off and on since early childhood. She also reported a tendency toward getting lost, much better verbal than arithmetic skills, no skill in drawing or singing, and trouble getting along with others. The latter was associated with shyness, which, in turn, was associated with trouble knowing how to manage routine social interactions.

Because this constellation of symptoms suggested right-hemisphere dysfunction, Sally was given a battery of neuropsychological tests to examine her underlying ability to process information. These tests revealed excellent verbal intelligence (verbal IQ = 126); impaired nonverbal skills (performance IQ = 88); attention deficits consistent with attention-deficit/hyperactivity disorder, predominantly inattentive type; and markedly impaired visual-spatial-organizational skills. In addition, even though Sally had a strong desire for friendships, her questionnaire data revealed a consistent pattern of impaired social competence and anxiety about social interactions.

Sally was treated with a combination of pharmacotherapy, behavioral psychotherapy, and social skills training, which resulted in complete resolution of her OCD symptoms. Because of the severity of her neurologically based social skills and visual-spatial-organizational deficits, Sally continued to have significant, though less severe, problems with social interactions at the conclusion of her treatment.

DSM-IV Diagnoses

Axis I: 300.3   Obsessive-Compulsive Disorder
           314.00   Attention-Deficit/Hyperactivity Disorder,
                     Predominantly Inattentive Type

Discussion

Several lines of evidence suggest that impaired right-hemisphere function is not uncommon in OCD patients. Hollander et al. reported that of 19 adults with OCD, 13 had four or more neurological "soft signs."[1] Denckla reported of 54 OCD patients, 45 had some positive neurological findings and, specifically, 8 had left hemisyndrome, a marker of right-hemisphere dysfunction of a cognitive nature. As Denckla describes it, a person with left hemisyndrome would grow up with an imbalance between normal verbal ability and impaired nonverbal orientation and perception of the environment.[2] Sally's difficulty with making decisions, her social skills deficits, and her visual-spatial-organizational deficits likely stem from these relative deficits in right- versus left-hemisphere functioning. In patients with this constellation of symptoms, neuropsychological testing can confirm the diagnosis of a right-hemisphere deficit syndrome and provide a useful guide to neurobehavioral treatment.

Case Presentation 33
Scatologically Scared

Derek, a 13-year-old, was sent to his school guidance counselor because he refused to attend school. After questioning Derek, the

---

[1]Hollander E, Schiffman E, Cohen B, et al.: "Signs of Central Nervous System Dysfunction in Obsessive-Compulsive Disorder." *Archives of General Psychiatry* 47:27–32, 1990.

[2]Denckla MB: "Neurological Examination," in *Obsessive-Compulsive Disorder in Children and Adolescents.* Edited by Rapoport JL. Washington, DC, American Psychiatric Press, 1989, pp. 107–115.

counselor was confused by his story and referred him for evaluation by a child psychiatrist. Derek's story was indeed confusing because his refusal to attend school was driven by the obsession, "Don't poop at school." His corresponding rituals entailed spending 3 or 4 hours defecating each morning before school and taking a constipating agent. At his first visit, Derek acknowledged that he was very much aware of the senseless nature of his symptoms but that he felt powerless to resist them. Derek had no other OCD symptoms and met criteria for no other DSM-IV disorder. The patient's family history was positive for OCD in his mother (as a child) and for major depressive disorder in his father. Derek responded well to an exposure and response-prevention regimen consisting of a return to school, use of the school bathrooms, discontinuation of the constipating agent, and cessation of his defecation rituals.

DSM-IV Diagnosis

Axis I: 300.3 Obsessive-Compulsive Disorder

Discussion

A few psychiatric syndromes—including hypochondriasis, body dysmorphic disorder, and somatization disorder—have symptoms so similar to those of OCD that diagnostic distinctions are not always clear. Derek's symptoms superficially resemble a specific social phobia, namely, social anxiety around defecating in a public place. However, careful questioning revealed that Derek's symptoms were driven by a very specific obsession rather than by social anxiety. Moreover, Derek found it impossible to resist his compulsions to empty his bowel and then put in a "plug," and he readily recognized the senselessness of his actions. Another clue to the diagnosis of OCD was the presence of a positive family history. Approximately 20% of children with OCD have a first-degree relative with the disorder; one-third of adults with OCD report that the onset of their OCD occurred by age 15.

Case Presentation 34
The Girl Who Couldn't Stop Spitting

Emily, an 8-year-old, was seen by her pediatrician because her mother was concerned that her daughter's need to spit into a paper towel or tissue "wasn't normal." Emily's mother also reported that Emily had "stopped eating" and had lost several pounds over the weeks preceding her visit. The pediatrician then referred Emily for consultation with a child psychiatrist to rule out anorexia nervosa.

During her interview, Emily reported a 3-month obsession with "germs in spit," which she feared might cause her to become ill if she swallowed her saliva. Emily was initially able to ignore the obsession but later began spitting to control the obsession and associated phobic anxiety about becoming ill. Her need to spit was increased by anything that increased the production of saliva; thus Emily also began avoiding food, especially spicy or sour foods. Although Emily recognized that her germ phobia was "different," she considered it sensible to be afraid of germs. Despite this loss of insight, she was quite embarrassed by her symptoms and only reluctantly revealed them to the examining physician. Emily met criteria for no DSM-IV disorder except OCD; her family history was negative for mental illness.

Emily responded to pharmacotherapy followed by an exposure and response-prevention regimen. This behavioral technique consists of "exposure" to the feared situation or substance (saliva, in this case) and help in resisting the urge to engage in compulsions (spitting, in this case) to reduce discomfort.

DSM-IV Diagnosis

Axis I: 300.3   Obsessive-Compulsive Disorder

Discussion

Upon superficial examination, Emily appeared to have an eating disorder, and, indeed, she did refuse to eat because of her obsessional fear of swallowing saliva. However, her symptoms lacked several of the cardinal features of anorexia nervosa, particularly an obsessional concern with thinness. Rather, her obsession was with contamination, and the resulting compulsion was to spit as a means of avoiding the "germs" that, she believed, were contained in saliva. This case illustrates the importance of a careful analysis of the symptom presentation of OCD. Such a precise phenomenological analysis is required for accurate diagnosis as well as for application of effective behavioral psychotherapy and pharmacotherapy.

Case Presentation 35
Fat or Thin? That Is the Question

Jeff, a 15-year-old with an obsessional fear of becoming fat, was hospitalized in an eating disorders unit, where he was being tube-fed because of his refusal to eat. In addition to avoiding food, Jeff also refused to touch "fat people" or even to touch things that "fat people" had touched for fear of gaining weight. Jeff had no desire for "thinness" per se and had never engaged in the kind of weight-loss strategies, such as purging or exercising, common to patients with anorexia nervosa. More important, Jeff found his obsessional thoughts and consequent rituals extremely unpleasant, stating clearly that he considered them "crazy" and "nonsense." When confronted by a psychodynamic interpretation of his chief symptom as "aggressive wishes toward his mother," Jeff told his psychotherapist, "You're crazier than I am."

Because of Jeff's confusing mixture of symptoms, consultation was requested and the correct diagnosis of OCD was made. Interestingly, a helpful clue to the diagnosis was given by his mother. She reminded Jeff about a variety of motor rituals he had forgotten about, including hand washing, that he had engaged in when he was 6 years old. Because these symptoms were transient, a diagnosis of OCD had not been made at that time. In addition, Jeff's family history on both sides was positive for OCD and affective disorder.

Jeff and his family were given a careful neurobehavioral explanation of OCD, and based on this understanding, they readily agreed to Jeff's participating in a combination of behavior therapy and pharmacotherapy. Tube feeding was discontinued, pharmacotherapy was initiated, and Jeff started a program of exposure and response prevention, consisting of eating and contact with "fat people." He rapidly began to resume normal eating behaviors and was soon discharged from the hospital.

DSM-IV Diagnosis

Axis I: 300.3   Obsessive-Compulsive Disorder

Discussion

This case illustrates well the importance of the clinician's making a careful phenomenological analysis when dealing with obsessional symptomatology superficially resembling an eating disorder. The patient lacked the intense wish to be thin that is one of the main clinical features of anorexia nervosa, as well as the weight-loss strategies so characteristic of this pursuit of thinness. Rather, he considered his obsessional thoughts about "fat people" and the consequent rituals "crazy" and nonsensical, although he could not resist them.

Case Presentation 36
Obsessed With OCD

Sharon, a 14-year-old, was scheduled by her mother, Mrs. P., for assessment in an outpatient clinic. During the initial phone screening, Mrs. P. told the clinic social worker that Sharon had OCD but that her daughter's condition had been misdiagnosed for many years. Mrs. P. wanted to be certain that her daughter would be seeing an expert in OCD, because her case was highly unusual and severe.

Because of her disability, Sharon had been placed in special education throughout her schooling and had never developed any close
peer relationships. Mrs. P. went on to describe how Sharon was
obsessed with the texture of certain objects, with the arrangement
of the furniture in the house, and with the order of her day-to-day
routine.

The social worker asked Mrs. P. if she would allow the clinic to
obtain records of Sharon's past treatment. Surprisingly, Mrs. P.
declined and was somewhat evasive about the reason. After closer
questioning, she admitted to extreme dissatisfaction with Sharon's
previous doctors because "they know nothing about obsessive-
compulsive disorder and don't understand Sharon at all." She went
on to say that Sharon was a gifted child and that few people
recognized her special talents. When the social worker asked if she
could contact the school for background material before the assessment, Mrs. P. again refused, insisting that the doctor have a "fresh,
unbiased perspective."

Sharon came to the assessment appointment with both of her
parents. During the interview, Mrs. P. did virtually all the talking
while her husband sat in uncomfortable silence. Sharon was very
neatly dressed and sat quietly on the couch beside her mother
without uttering a word. Throughout the interview, she never spoke
but looked completely composed and relaxed as she rhythmically
stroked a satin ribbon on her dress.

The doctor began the interview by asking simply, "What is it
about Sharon that concerns you?" Mrs. P. then described how
Sharon had been unusual since birth and that she had been taken
to many doctors, all of whom were baffled. Mrs. P. said that she had
seen a popular television show featuring an expert on OCD who
described behaviors that were "identical to Sharon's." Mrs. P. then
read everything she could find about OCD, which confirmed her
impression that this disorder was indeed at the root of Sharon's
problems.

When the doctor asked specifically what sort of abnormal
behaviors Sharon actually exhibited, Mrs. P. described how Sharon
was very obsessed with the texture of certain items. She said, "See
how she's stroking that ribbon; you can see she's obsessed. If I didn't
stop her, she would sit there and stroke that ribbon just like that all

day long." Meanwhile Sharon seemed completely oblivious to the discussion and continued to rub the ribbon. Her mother went on to describe how Sharon would shriek and scream uncontrollably if even one piece of furniture was out of place in the household. She said that Sharon would simply not stop screaming until the furniture was restored to its original location. In addition, Sharon had to complete her morning dressing ritual in a very specific way that was exactly the same each day. Any deviations from this routine resulted in more screaming and temper tantrums.

When the doctor asked about Sharon's intellectual and motor development, Mrs. P. explained that Sharon was a very intelligent child, perhaps even a genius. During this part of the interview, Sharon's father seemed especially uncomfortable. When the doctor asked Mrs. P. to elaborate, she explained that Sharon had an extraordinary memory and knew every family member and every acquaintance by their automobile license plate number. When family or friends would come to visit, Sharon would immediately recite their license plate number and the make and model of their car. Mrs. P. explained that this meant that Sharon was actually very intelligent despite the fact she had made little academic progress in school. Mrs. P. found it particularly galling that the school seemed to view Sharon's intellectual development as delayed and had placed her in classrooms for persons with mental retardation.

During part of the assessment, Sharon was interviewed alone. She did not seem the least concerned when her parents left the room and simply continued to stroke the satin ribbon on her dress. When the doctor asked Sharon questions, she did not seem to respond in any way and appeared to be avoiding eye contact. When the doctor attempted to interrupt her ribbon-stroking behavior, she immediately screamed "No, no, no!" and grabbed the ribbon back. At no time did Sharon acknowledge the doctor as a person or develop any meaningful rapport.

At the conclusion of the assessment, the doctor met with Sharon's parents to give them his initial impressions. He said gently but firmly, "It is extremely unlikely that your daughter has obsessive-compulsive disorder. Instead I think she has a disorder called autism."

Mrs. P. then burst into tears while her husband gave the doctor a knowing look and rolled his eyes. After weeping quietly for several minutes, Mrs. P. composed herself, graciously thanked the doctor for his time, and left with Sharon and her husband. When contacted by clinic staff about completing the evaluation, Mrs. P. politely refused, saying, "We plan to take Sharon elsewhere."

DSM-IV Diagnosis

Axis I: None
Axis II· 299.00   Autistic Disorder

Discussion

Autistic disorder and OCD superficially share several characteristics. In both disorders, patients engage in repetitive, stereotypic behaviors and often appear very anxious. However, patients with OCD are usually normal in most other respects, whereas patients with autism typically exhibit abnormal behavior in almost all aspects of their lives. Like most patients with autism, Sharon exhibited a bizarre lack of interpersonal relatedness, had language and other communication deficits, and had mental retardation. Although OCD and autism share some superficial similarities, they are so distinct that experienced clinicians have little difficulty differentiating one disorder from the other.

Mrs. P. had still not come to terms with the painful fact of having a developmentally disabled child. Her intense desire to have a more normal daughter made Mrs. P. fixate on the notion that Sharon was suffering from OCD. Although she was initially upset by the diagnosis of probable autism, Mrs. P. later told clinic personnel that the doctor was a nice man but too young and inexperienced to make a correct diagnosis.

CME Test
Chapter 6
Case Presentations 31–36

Please read the six sets of questions (12 questions total) that follow and circle the one best answer for each question on the corresponding answer sheet in the accompanying booklet.

Case Presentation 31: Compulsive Cutting

31A. This patient's ability to resist her urges to harm herself stems from which one of the following factors?

1 The combination of pharmacotherapy and exposure and response-prevention treatment initiated when her obsessive-compulsive disorder (OCD) was diagnosed.
2. Her perception of the entire obsessional experience as ego-dystonic.
3. Her ability to avoid knives and other sharp items.

31B. In this patient's case, her urges to cut herself and her subsequent avoidance of knives and razors seem to be best associated with which one of the following histories?

1. Previous sexual or physical abuse with related Axis II psychopathology.
2. Childhood compulsions in response to obsessions that she recognized but could do nothing about.
3. Suppressed desires to communicate a complex mixture of revenge and dependency needs.

Case Presentation 32: Shopping for the Number 4

32A. Which of the following statements best describes the frequency of occurrence of right-hemispheric dysfunction in patients with OCD?

1. It never occurs.
2. It is rare.
3. It is not uncommon.

32B. This patient's continuing social-skills deficits most probably stem from which one of the following factors?

1. Her OCD.
2. Her impaired right-hemisphere functioning.
3. Her concern with the number 4.

Case Presentation 33: Scatologically Scared

33A. Which one of the following factors best differentiated this patient's diagnosis of OCD from syndromes with similar symptoms, such as delusional disorder, somatic?

1. His obsession about not defecating at school.
2. His compulsive use of a constipating agent to lessen obsessional anxiety about defecating at school.
3. His recognition of the senselessness of his actions.

33B. What is the approximate percentage of children diagnosed with OCD who have a first-degree relative with the disorder?

1. 60%
2. 15%
3. 20%

Case Presentation 34: The Girl Who Couldn't Stop Spitting

34A. Anorexia nervosa was ruled out in this patient's case. Which one of the following considerations helped to eliminate that diagnosis?

1. She recognized and was embarrassed by her symptoms.
2. She lacked an obsessional concern with thinness.
3. She was obsessed with contamination.

34B. The phenomenological analysis of this patient's presentation of OCD symptoms was best aided by which one of the following factors?

1. She avoided spicy foods to decrease her saliva output.
2. She showed an obsession with contamination and felt compelled to expel "germs" in her saliva by spitting.

3. Her "eating disorder" resulted in OCD marked by spitting and a refusal to eat.

Case Presentation 35: Fat or Thin? That Is the Question

35A. The patient was hospitalized in an eating disorders unit, where he was being tube-fed because of his refusal to eat. Why was an eating disorder not a diagnosis in this case?

1. Weight-loss strategies characteristic of the pursuit of thinness were not present in this patient.
2. His confusing mix of symptoms precluded a diagnosis of an eating disorder.
3. His avoidance of "fat people" and things they had touched was not compatible with such a diagnosis.

35B. What reinforces the diagnosis of OCD in this case?

1. The patient's refusal to touch "fat people."
2. The patient's mother's recounting of his variety of motor rituals at age 6.
3. The patient's "aggressive wishes toward his mother."

Case Presentation 36: Obsessed With OCD

36A. The physician concluded that this patient was autistic. Which one of the following features of the patient's behavior best helps to confirm the physician's diagnosis?

1. Her stereotypic repetitive behaviors (e.g., ribbon stroking).
2. Her level of anxiety (e.g., refusal to release her ribbon).
3. Her impairment in reciprocal social interaction (e.g., her inability to acknowledge the doctor or to develop any meaningful rapport).

36B. After expressed dissatisfaction with previous doctors, the patient's mother refused to acknowledge this most recent physician's diagnosis of autism and maintained that her daughter suffered from OCD, presumably because

1. The patient's compulsive acts (e.g., ribbon stroking) were a dominant feature of her behavior.

2. Of her inability to accept that her daughter had a profoundly severe disorder often associated with mental retardation.
3. Her daughter exhibited genius-level intelligence.

Case Presentation 37
Panic in the Sealed Room

Alan, a 47-year-old, has been divorced for 7 years. He is well dressed and groomed, and his manner is pleasant and cooperative. Alan is an Israeli schoolmaster who has been referred to therapy for "panic attacks" he experienced during the Persian Gulf War. Several times during the war when an alert for an Iraqi missile attack was announced, Israeli residents were required to enter a sealed room and stay there, wearing gas masks for several hours. Alan experienced severe anxiety in the sealed room and refused to wear his gas mask throughout the war. He says that the sealed room made him feel as if he were choking, just as he had first felt when at age 19 he had had to work in a bunker during his military service. Alan says he has similar feelings, on a smaller scale, when riding the bus, sitting in a movie theater, or entering a cave with his pupils, and he tends to avoid these situations. Fear of enclosed places prevents him from driving his car far away from home at night; darkness then seems to "close in" on him.

Alan describes himself as obsessive and a perfectionist. He constantly worries about his work. How is he going to secure money for needed renovations? Is he going to make the deadline for absorbing new pupils? He also describes himself as being "crazy" about cleanliness, a trait that was a source of bitter arguments with his former wife. At his insistence, he and his wife spent many hours ironing, laundering clothes, and mopping the floors and walls. He still performs these chores even though he has regularly scheduled hired help. He cleans the kitchen himself daily, in addition to cleaning the entire apartment three times a week. Alan says he "cannot stand dirt," and if he sees a speck of dust on the rug, he feels compelled to pick it up.

Cleaning gives Alan a sense of control over his life. Control is an important issue for him: he has a hard time coping with uncertainty and conflict. He is self-reliant, demands a lot from himself and others, and has a hard time trusting anyone else to do things just right. He is very efficient, tends to follow his own strict "principles" and "rules," and is extremely devoted to his work. Alan has difficulties in interpersonal relationships, and others describe him as cold and rigid. Alan gets upset when things do not go his way, and he tends to impose his will on co-workers and family. For example, he recently insisted that his severely depressed daughter attend a family wedding despite her reluctance, telling her categorically that "everyone should come to these family events."

DSM-IV Diagnoses

Axis I: 300.29   Specific Phobia, Situational Type
Axis II: 301.4   Obsessive-Compulsive Personality Disorder

Discussion

Does Alan have obsessive-compulsive disorder (OCD)? The diagnostic criteria for OCD require the presence of either obsessions or compulsions. Although Alan sees himself as obsessive, he does not report ideas, thoughts, impulses, or images that he experiences as intrusive and senseless; rather, his worries about his work are apparently ego-syntonic. His cleaning, though it follows strict rules and seems excessive, is not directly designed to neutralize discomfort and is not, for the most part, experienced as unreasonable. Rather, it seems a part of a perfectionistic, rigid, and rule-oriented way of life. Alan is a person preoccupied with rules and order, insisting that others submit to his way of doing things and not trusting others to do things right. He has difficulty expressing warm feelings, and his devotion to work dominates his life and precludes intimate interpersonal relationships. This pattern clearly meets the criteria for obsessive-compulsive personality disorder rather than OCD.

In addition, Alan's difficulty in and avoidance of enclosed spaces, which culminated in his experience in the sealed room, warrants a diagnosis of specific phobia, situational type (claustrophobia). Agoraphobia might also be considered because of Alan's report of feeling trapped when he enters a cave or sits on a bus or in a theater, where a graceful and speedy exit would be difficult.

Case Presentation 38
"I Love Him—I Love Him Not"

Pat is a pale and slender 24-year-old woman with long, straight hair. She speaks rapidly and nervously and cries often during her intake session. She says that she has always dreamed of having a boyfriend and now she does—his name is Steven. But things are not going well: she has been suffering from unrelenting, nagging doubts about their relationship.

Pat met Steven 4 months ago through a female friend of hers. He has had several girlfriends before; for her, the relationship is a first, and Steven is the only man with whom she has ever had a sexual relationship. Pat began to have doubts when they first spoke of love only 2 months after meeting. She told Steven she was not yet sure she knew what love was, and he replied that he thought he had taught her *that* since they met. She went home and could not stop thinking about their discussion. She wondered whether she really did love him or whether she was going out with him only because she wanted a boyfriend.

Pat has continued to have such thoughts. She realizes that Steven does not really meet her ideal. He is not really handsome, for instance. They do not have common interests: he loves sports and heavy metal music, which she does not care for. He is neither romantic nor considerate enough. She wonders whether she should leave him and search for her "prince" or whether she can resolve her doubts and love him the way he is. She has crying spells at home, wishing for an answer, wanting to feel that she loves Steven. These obsessive doubts keep flooding Pat's consciousness "day and night." They come into her mind without warning, out of context, even in the midst of a telephone conversation with a friend.

Interestingly, Pat's frequent arguments with Steven are quite different in character from her obsessions about him. She demands that he tell her he loves her, that he say he would be willing to marry her right now. She interrogates him about his previous girlfriends and compares herself with them. She is especially preoccupied with Sally, who apparently "could read Steven's mind and did not have to be told what to do in bed." Pat, in contrast, acts, as Steven described to her, "like a mechanical doll." When Pat and Steven talk about sex, she feels that she is not good at it. She wishes she were as good as Sally. If she were good in bed, she could somehow resolve her "love–don't love" conflict.

Pat says that she has lost her appetite and has had a difficult time falling asleep in the past several weeks. Sometimes she wakes up in the middle of the night visualizing Sally and Steven in bed. At such moments, she is flooded with obsessions and tears.

Pat was born with a slight hearing difficulty, which made her participation in class and social activities difficult and impaired her school performance. She has always been extremely shy and lonely. She would join social activities in school, with considerable doubt and fear, but would then "just sit there like a mummy." She almost never spoke in class for fear that she would get confused and say something stupid. Although she tried her best to do as well as her peers, she "just barely" finished high school. After high school she stayed at home and has never worked. She has been reluctant to go to college, feeling she would never be able to study hard enough. At home she carries much of the burden, because her mother is busy at work. Pat takes housework seriously and is very particular ("sterile" is her word) about cleanliness and order. She continues to be afraid to be with people and has only one close friend, the woman who introduced her to Steven.

DSM-IV Diagnosis

Axis I: None
Axis II: 301.82   Avoidant Personality Disorder

Discussion

Pat complains of malignant doubts, which clearly cause marked distress and are time-consuming. Are these true obsessions? Does she suffer from OCD? DSM-IV criteria demand that obsessions be experienced, at least initially, as intrusive and senseless and that there be an attempt to ignore, suppress, or neutralize them. Pat's ruminations do not have these qualities. Instead, Pat's constant doubts about her feelings toward Steven seem a thin disguise for her deep-rooted doubts about her own adequacy. Although she is obsessed with the question of whether she loves Steven or whether he is good enough for her, one gets the clear impression that she is, in fact, questioning whether she is good enough—whether she can meet Steven's standards and expectations. This hypothesis is corroborated by Pat's history of social isolation, fear of rejection and embarrassment, reticence in social situations, and extremely low self-esteem. The pervasive pattern of social discomfort, fear of negative evaluation, and timidity meets the DSM-IV criteria for avoidant personality disorder.

Case Presentation 39
OCD in the Guise of Alcohol Abuse

A 38-year-old mother of two teenage boys was brought to the hospital with a history of excessive drinking for about a month. Norma had been found lying on the kitchen floor in a drunken state, which led to the visit to the emergency room. Her husband was so upset that he did not want anything to do with her. She was desperate, saying that her life was very depressing and riddled with anxiety. The only way she could make herself feel better was to drink so much that she did not know what was going on. "I hate the taste of alcohol," Norma confided, "but drinking is the only way for me to forget about things." Preliminary questions revealed nothing depressing in her environment. Her husband was financially well off and was a caring person. Their two children were doing well.

Upon further questioning, Norma revealed that the source of her anxiety and depression was the constant intrusion of the idea that she might have breast cancer. She knew very well that she enjoyed good health. She tried to push aside the idea that she had breast cancer, but it constantly intruded, and her anxiety continued to mount. When the anxiety became intolerable, she would call different gynecologists to get mammograms. She had had over 30 mammograms during the past 2 years.

A mental status examination revealed the presence of a dominant obsession about breast cancer and the compulsion to get mammograms. The patient did not have the classic symptoms of depression.

DSM-IV Diagnoses

Axis I: 300.3   Obsessive-Compulsive Disorder
           305.00   Alcohol Abuse

Discussion

What apparently disturbs Norma most is the constant intrusion of certain ideas related to her health that force themselves into her awareness against her will. These thoughts have all the characteristics of obsessions: they are recurrent and persistent, and even though she recognizes them as products of her own mind (she knows she enjoys good health), the anxiety builds until she is compelled to arrange for a mammogram. Because Norma's obsessions cause her marked distress and do not seem to be related to her interpretation of actual or perceived physical signs and sensations as evidence of physical illness, a diagnosis of OCD rather than hypochondriasis is warranted. A differential distinction must also be made between OCD and delusional disorder of the somatic type. In this case, the patient can acknowledge, at least to a certain extent, that the fear is unfounded, and hence it is not a delusion. Finally, it should be mentioned that sometimes hypochondriasis and OCD with somatic obsessions do not separate neatly.

Case Presentation 40
A Case of Schizophrenia?

A 25-year-old woman, Margaret, was brought to the hospital by her husband with the complaint that she was "a schizophrenic." The husband described her as having two personalities. She was like an animal at certain times and was a loving and caring wife at others.

History revealed that the patient was normal through her late teens and did well in school. She finished 2 years of college and started working as a secretary. Around age 21, Margaret began to feel compelled to bark like a dog. She felt stupid that this idea would jump into her head periodically, and she was able to control the compulsion to bark with some resulting anxiety.

A few years later the patient married, and she and her husband moved to an apartment. The initial stress of married life made her anxious, and the result was that she actually did bark like a dog once in a while. This behavior created problems. Because Margaret's husband was a salesman, he entertained clients on a regular basis, but he was unable to take his new wife to dinner with him for fear of embarrassment. Moreover, the couple was asked to leave four different apartments because of barking incidents. Consequently, Margaret became depressed—she was making her husband miserable and did not understand why such a ridiculous idea came into her head. She also felt compelled to shout uncontrollably on various occasions.

On physical examination Margaret exhibited "shoulder shrugs" that she reported had been present since childhood.

DSM-IV Diagnosis

Axis I: 307.23   Tourette's Disorder

Discussion

Tourette's disorder is frequently associated with OCD. An interesting phenomenological similarity between the two disorders is the partial control that most patients are able to exert over their seemingly involuntary symptoms, as is the case with this patient. In a published, subjective account, one patient described the movements and vocalizations of Tourette's disorder as desperate attempts to resolve a "psychic itch" that builds into unbearable torture unless the tension is released through the voluntary action of the symptom.[1] Even those who consider the nature of Tourette's symptoms "involuntary" acknowledge that the release of tension may be postponed with sufficient motivation or distraction.[2] In OCD a similar process seems to occur. In fact, the disorder is partially defined by the ego-dystonic nature of the obsessions and compulsions themselves and by the distress and mounting tension they induce when the person attempts to resist them.

A major difference between the two disorders appears to be the greater complexity of the cognitive structures governing obsessive-compulsive symptomatic actions. Also, Tourette's disorder is much less common in females than in males, and the average age at onset is 7 years, well before 20, the average age at onset of OCD. Whether the late age at onset (i.e., 21 years) of Tourette's in Margaret's case suggests a specific insult to the basal ganglia or the late emergence of a familial disorder could be addressed, in part, by a careful determination of the patient's family history of any tics or obsessions and compulsions.

[1] Cohen AJ, Leckman JF: "Sensory Phenomena Associated With Gilles de la Tourette's Syndrome." *Journal of Clinical Psychiatry* 53:319–323, 1992.

[2] Shapiro AK, Shapiro ES, Young JG, et al.: *Gilles de la Tourette Syndrome*. New York, Raven, 1988.

In light of the substantial percentage of patients with comorbid Tourette's disorder and OCD (46% to 90%), this patient was evaluated for OCD, as well as Tourette's. From both a clinical evaluation and the results of the Yale-Brown Obsessive Compulsive Checklist and Scale and the Maudsley Obsessive-Compulsive Inventory, it was determined that the patient did not meet the criteria for OCD. The diagnosis of Tourette's disorder was made, based on her history of vocal tics (barking, in this case) and on motor tics she exhibited during physical examination.

Case Presentation 41
The Epileptic Adolescent With
Obsessive-Compulsive Symptoms

Earl, a 14-year-old, was brought to the hospital because of compulsions that prevented him from leaving his room. Since the age of 5 years, the patient had been suffering from epilepsy characterized by grand mal seizures that occurred about once a week. The patient did not have any particular aura but manifested postepileptic confusion for 2 to 3 hours. He was treated daily with an antiepileptic drug. There was a history of forceps delivery, but Earl had done well in school, and his intelligence apparently had not been affected.

When Earl was 12 years old, he developed a number of compulsive behaviors. He insisted on sleeping facing east so that upon waking he would see the sun's rays. He would climb out of bed and then stand in front of his bed performing rituals for 3 to 5 minutes. From there he would proceed to the bathroom, where he would wash his fingers in a particular order a certain number of times. By the age of 13, Earl would get out of bed only if his sheets were arranged in a particular way and the window curtains were open such that the rays of the sun fell on the floor and not on his bed. When awakened, he would sit on his bed, requiring a male member of the family to stand on his right and a female on his left, both wearing white clothes. These family members had to remain in place until he went into the bathroom, which he would not do until the sun's rays fell on his face. He ate in his room and did not touch any strangers for fear of contamination. Eventually the fear of contamination and the complexity of the rituals prevented Earl from leaving his room at all.

As a result of these compulsions, the patient's family brought him to the hospital for evaluation. An electroencephalogram (EEG) confirmed earlier diagnoses and showed that a left temporal lobe focus had emerged. Antiepileptic drug therapy was reevaluated, and the resulting regimen was more effective in suppressing seizures. However, Earl's rituals continued unabated and became more elaborate in the hospital setting.

DSM-IV Diagnoses

Axis I: 300.3   Obsessive-Compulsive Disorder
Axis II: None
Axis III: Epilepsy

Discussion

Earl has a clear-cut history of epilepsy, characterized by tonic-clonic (grand mal) seizures that had not been well controlled with medication. Many years after the onset of epilepsy, he developed disabling obsessive-compulsive symptoms. The diagnosis of OCD was difficult. There can be clinical similarities between patients with temporal lobe epilepsy and those with OCD. For example, several authors have described "involuntary forced thinking" in patients with temporal lobe epilepsy as documented by EEG evidence.[3] In contrast to epilepsy patients, patients with OCD are usually aware that their obsessions and compulsions are excessive or unreasonable and recognize them as products of their own minds.[4] The patient in this case, however, did not demonstrate such clear awareness.

---

[3] Jenike MA: "Theories of Etiology," in *Obsessive-Compulsive Disorders: Theory and Management*, 2nd Edition. Edited by Jenike MA, Baer L, Minichiello WE. Chicago, IL, Year Book Medical, 1990.

[4] Engel J: *Seizures and Epilepsy*. Philadelphia, PA, FA Davis, 1989, p. 354.

In the final analysis, the diagnosis of OCD was made, and Earl responded well to pharmacotherapy.

Case Presentation 42
Mother's Backache Reveals the
Patient With OCD

Upon the advice of physicians, a 41-year-old, single, unemployed man was brought to the hospital by his mother for psychiatric evaluation. Henry had been living with and been dependent on his 68-year-old mother for years. Nine months before his arrival at the clinic, the patient developed a recurrence of severe and incapacitating symptoms precipitated by watching a television show in which an elderly woman was killed. After watching the show, whenever Henry heard a certain word(s) on television that meant "death" or "dying," he would then recite the word(s) 16 times and promptly write it down on paper. He would then instruct his mother to repeat certain phrases having to do with "actions," such as "go to the market," "go to the store," "go to the bank," and so forth. Following this recitation, he would ask his mother to repeat the word(s) related to death or dying 16 times and then again once or twice. Next, he would instruct his mother to repeat action-oriented sentences unrelated to what was said previously, such as, "It is time to eat." "brush your teeth." "wash your face." "comb your hair." As his mother recited the sentences, the son would remain tense and motionless, counting the number of times each sentence was recited. After these rituals were completed, Henry would scan the room closely to make sure everything was in order. His mother would reluctantly perform the rituals to help relieve her son's anxiety. Because she had to stand for long periods of time during each recitation, the mother developed a backache, which led her to seek treatment at the hospital, where she was advised to bring her son in for treatment.

DSM-IV Diagnosis

Axis I: 300.3   Obsessive-Compulsive Disorder

Discussion

The devastating impact that severe OCD can have on family functioning is apparent in this case presentation. In this instance, the mother, as well as the son, had become victim to the disorder. What makes this case especially poignant is the emotional blackmail practiced by Henry on his mother in convincing her that his anxiety could be relieved only by her behavior. Livingston-Van Noppen and colleagues have observed that the three most common family response patterns to OCD are characterized as "enmeshed," "antagonistic," and "split."[5] Clearly, the mother in this case is thoroughly enmeshed in her son's rituals in an effort to keep peace and reduce anxiety. Family-system therapists discourage this type of overinvolved behavior because it contributes to the deterioration of social and occupational functioning of the affected person. Behavior therapists also discourage family participation in rituals because such participation aggravates rather than relieves the disorder.

[5]Livingston-Van Noppen B, Rasmussen SA, Eisen J, et al.: "Family Function and Treatment in OCD," in *Obsessive-Compulsive Disorders: Theory and Management*, 2nd Edition. Edited by Jenike MA, Baer L, Minichiello WE. Chicago, IL, Year Book Medical, 1990, pp. 325–340.

CME Test
Chapter 7
Case Presentations 37–42

Please read the six sets of questions (12 questions total) that follow and circle the one best answer for each question on the corresponding answer sheet in the accompanying booklet.

Case Presentation 37: Panic in the Sealed Room

37A. Among the indications that the patient in this case does *not* have obsessive-compulsive disorder (OCD) is that

1. He is obsessed with the idea of control.
2. His need to keep his apartment clean, although possibly excessive, is not experienced by him as unreasonable.
3. He is afraid of enclosed spaces.

37B. Which of the following symptom clusters in this patient most clearly points to the diagnosis of obsessive-compulsive personality disorder (OCPD)?

1. Extreme devotion to work, difficulty in delegating tasks, difficulty in expressing affection.
2. Fear of darkness "closing in," cleaning rituals, controlling personality.
3. Difficulty coping with conflict, ego-syntonic obsession with cleanliness, avoidance of enclosed places.

Case Presentation 38: "I Love Him—I Love Him Not"

30A. The patient's ruminations about her significant other

1. Reflect her low self-esteem.
2. Are both senseless and intrusive.
3. Prevent her from enjoying a normal sex life.

38B. A trait characteristic of avoidant personality disorder and exhibited by the patient in this case is

1. A hearing deficit.

2. A history of social isolation.
3. Frequent arguments with significant others.

Case Presentation 39: OCD in the Guise of Alcohol Abuse

39A. One indication that the patient in this case is not presenting with hypochondriasis is that

1. She does not seek a new physician each time she has a mammogram.
2. She acknowledges that she enjoys good health.
3. She exhibits classic symptoms of depression.

39B. Which is true of the patient's fear of breast cancer?

1. It is apparently unrelated to her abuse of alcohol.
2. It suggests that she may have a delusional disorder.
3. It makes her so anxious at times that she feels compelled to have repeated mammograms.

Case Presentation 40: A Case of Schizophrenia?

40A. One distinction between OCD and Tourette's disorder is

1. The average age at onset, which is earlier in Tourette's disorder.
2. Tourette's disorder is equally common in men and women.
3. The cognitive structures that govern symptomatic actions in OCD are less complex than those that govern Tourette's disorder.

40B. Which of the following is true of the patient's compulsion to bark?

1. It is a vocal tic.
2. She has no control over the barking.
3. It is a conscious ritual.

Case Presentation 41: The Epileptic Adolescent With Obsessive-Compulsive Symptoms

41A. Which of the following accounts for the clinician's difficulty in diagnosing OCD in this case?

1. The patient is clearly aware that his rituals are unreasonable.

2. Involuntary, forced thinking may be associated with temporal lobe epilepsy as well as with OCD.
3. The patient's compulsions are masked by frequent grand mal seizures.

41B. The patient's compulsive behavior
   1. Was so extreme that his family took him to the hospital for evaluation.
   2. Was unaffected by pharmacotherapy.
   3. Began shortly after he was told he had epilepsy.

Case Presentation 42: Mother's Backache Reveals the Patient With OCD

42A. In this case, the mother's participation in her son's rituals
   1. Would be frowned upon by both family system and behavior therapists.
   2. Represents the split pattern of family response to OCD.
   3. Reflects the mother's fear of dying, which developed after her son saw a television show in which an elderly woman was killed.

42B. The son's ritualistic behavior in this case
   1. Is not typical of the compulsive behavior of patients with OCD.
   2. Has produced hypochondriasis in his mother.
   3. Is triggered by references to death or dying that he hears on television.

Case Presentation 43
The Circumnavigator

In response to the clinician's initial query regarding the reason for his consultation, Gus replied, "Dr. Stewart asked me to see you; he thought that you could help." Gus had been seeing his therapist for more than 10 years. Dr. Stewart had become a father figure, infallible but apparently not omnipotent. Gus had not benefited from 10 years of insight-oriented therapy and the occasional prescription of tranquilizers.

Gus was not psychotic, although his shallow affect and emotional withdrawal would raise the suspicions of even a novice mental health professional. He showed little spontaneity, seemed worried, and was mildly agitated. Often Gus would readjust his glasses; periodically he would wring his sweaty palms, and he was clearly hypervigilant. His "story" was going to be very difficult to tell.

"My mother is tired of it . . . I am almost 36 . . . I should not have to drag her everywhere I go." He told the story of a series of compulsions about symmetry and exactness beginning during early childhood at about the time of his father's death. His adult concerns were principally about driving, especially alone. There were so many cars; so many traffic lights, signs, and noises; so many decisions. A distraction, a distant siren, crossing an intersection as the light turned yellow, grazing the curb, or being slightly jolted by a bump were all causes to turn the car around and "check"—check that he had not struck or run over a pedestrian or caused another car to veer off the road and have an accident. Gus would turn the car around, again and again.

Having his mother in the car was a relief to Gus but not a solution. She was occasionally able to convince Gus not to turn the car around, but his disorder was now so severe that her reassurances were seldom enough. Gus recognized that he totally monopolized his mother's life. She accompanied him to his office almost daily, and yet he was still always late.

Gus had other compulsions. Parking in his building's garage was always troublesome. Beside the elevator, an ever-present sentinel greeted him. It was the pay phone, perched on its low pedestal. He was uncertain whether or not it would ring as the elevator door closed. Gus would ride the elevator several times until he was convinced that the phone was not ringing. The authorities could be calling him to accuse him of causing an accident or injuring a pedestrian on his way to work.

Once Gus crossed the threshold of his office, most of these irrational concerns vanished. At work, he was ambitious and efficient. He did not take breaks or attend any work-related functions. Contact with others made him uncomfortable even though, at the same time, he despised his secludedness. After almost 6 years with his firm, he had no friends. Yet he had an enviable cadre of affluent customers, always loyal because of his accurate investment forecasting.

The drive home was easier. He seldom checked, even though the obsessions of doom were always there. While his mother prepared dinner he would glance over the many work-related publications he had brought home. After dinner he would study them to prepare for the next day. Weekends were an opportunity to read an even larger volume of material or to enjoy the modern spy thrillers that provided him some escape. Because his father had been deceased since Gus was 6, Gus afforded his mother good company. He was celibate and had never risked a real date.

DSM-IV Diagnoses

Axis I: 300.3   Obsessive-Compulsive Disorder
Axis II: 301.82   Avoidant Personality Disorder

Discussion

The diagnostic combination of obsessive-compulsive disorder (OCD) and avoidant personality disorder is not uncommonly seen in clinical practice. Compulsions with symmetry and exactness that emerge in childhood can later lead to "checking." Patients of this type receive the message early from family and friends that they are peculiar, and these patients suffer silently from the ridicule of others. Their response is to withdraw from society while immersing themselves in specific activities or a fantasy world. Because of their aloofness, lack of spontaneity, and social isolation, they are often suspected by physicians of being psychotic. Yet, like Gus, they can be successful in highly competitive environments, even while exhibiting a pervasive pattern of social discomfort and avoidance. Therefore, although Gus had no close friends or confidant(e)s other than his mother and he avoided all social activities, he functioned well in his career because no significant interpersonal contact was required. A facilitative, knowledgeable therapist can uncover symptoms of both OCD and avoidant personality disorder and begin appropriate behavioral, pharmacological, and psychotherapeutic management.

Case Presentation 44
His Family's Shame

Dr. Holden, an experienced therapist, urged a colleague to consult with one of his patients, Greg. Dr. Holden shared little with his colleague about the patient other than the belief that Greg had OCD.

Greg called the consulting psychiatrist within a few days. The phone conversation was brief but revealing. Greg was 38, single, and unemployed. He lived with his parents and had seen Dr. Holden only twice. The patient told the psychiatrist that Dr. Holden had made a diagnosis of OCD. The initial telephone conversation was more like an interrogation, because Greg volunteered no information. Under close questioning, Greg revealed that he had first noticed his symptoms during early adolescence but did not know what he had. Greg added, "I have a sickness of rituals and doubts . . . My condition causes me phobias, extreme nervousness, and fears of having an accident or injuring someone." Greg's complaints seemed typical of persons with OCD.

A few days later the consulting psychiatrist met Greg. He was tall, at least 6′5″, and lanky. He appeared withdrawn and showed no spontaneity when the psychiatrist first greeted him. Greg walked slowly and deliberately into the psychiatrist's office. In a monotonous tone he shared his symptoms. Within a few minutes he told the psychiatrist about various rituals he performed, including checking, hoarding, and ordering compulsions. He also reported obsessions with contamination and being "tyrannized" by his doubts. Greg's affect was flat and he made no eye contact. It was as though he had memorized and rehearsed general descriptions of OCD from a textbook.

During his initial monologue it became clear that Greg was psychotic. As the interview proceeded, he reported ideas of reference and auditory hallucinations. He was also troubled by thought insertion and probably thought broadcasting. Surprisingly, he denied a history of previous psychiatric treatment and affirmed that his first evaluation had been by Dr. Holden.

With Greg's permission, the psychiatrist consulted with his sister by telephone a few days later, and it was then that the real story began to unfold. Apparently she, and perhaps others in the family, had "coached" Greg to report and focus on his obsessive-compulsive symptoms during his visit. The psychiatrist learned that Greg had been in and out of treatment in public facilities for a psychotic disorder since the age of 19.

DSM-IV Diagnosis

Axis I: 295.90   Schizophrenia, Undifferentiated Type

Discussion

Media attention to OCD has increased during the last few years. Many families long haunted by the distress and stigma of mental illness in a family member have hoped that the obsessive-compulsive symptoms that can accompany psychotic disorders would provide the long-awaited "answer" that leads to a cure. Indeed, many psychotic patients have obsessions about persecution and atypical and bizarre compulsive rituals, but obsessive-compulsive symptoms do not "make" the diagnosis of OCD. Although patients with OCD frequently have irrational or bizarre thoughts about their symptoms, they remain in touch with reality in other areas of their lives. For this reason, OCD is not considered to be a psychotic disorder. Greg had absolutely no insight into his illness.

The relationship between OCD and schizophrenia has not been resolved. Some authorities believe that OCD occasionally evolves into schizophrenia; others suggest that they are two different illnesses that sometimes coexist by chance. This latter concept is supported by a report of three sets of monozygotic twins who were concordant for OCD but discordant for schizophrenia and schizo-affective disorder.[1] Finally, evidence has been presented to suggest that OCD itself may take on psychotic features that in turn can result in a misdiagnosis of schizophrenia.[2]

Case Presentation 45
The Man Who Feared Particles

Thomas, a 65-year-old retired farmer, describes a 1-year history of fears that "particles" would enter his body and cause him to become ill. He is not obsessed with germs or infection but rather that he might inhale or swallow particulate materials from a great number of sources or that particles might become stuck in his throat or eye.

---

[1] Lewis SW, Chitkara B, Reveley AM: "Obsessive-Compulsive Disorder and Schizophrenia in Three Identical Twin Pairs." *Psychological Medicine* 21:135–141, 1991.

[2] Insel TR, Akiskal HS: "Obsessive-Compulsive Disorder With Psychotic Features: A Phenomenologic Analysis." *American Journal of Psychiatry* 143:1527–1533, 1986.

He has consulted numerous doctors, complaining of the sensation of a foreign body in his throat or in his eye or elsewhere in his body. Even though he has undergone numerous physical examinations, Thomas has failed to respond to the numerous reassurances that he is normal.

The sound of two bottles "clinking" together is a sign of danger to Thomas because of the possibility that a minute glass particle might have become dislodged, with him as the target. Passing through a doorway is always a risk because particles might rub off the door frame and contaminate him. He once left a restaurant before finishing his meal when he saw a workman change a light bulb— a sure indication that particles would drop into his food. In an attempt to avoid particles, he always wipes his silverware and closely scrutinizes all surfaces of his dinnerware before eating. While seated in the interviewer's office, Thomas suddenly moves to another chair when he realizes that the one he had been occupying is located directly under a ceiling air vent—another source of dreaded particles. When in public, he keeps his mouth closed as much as possible, allowing his nose to filter potentially dangerous particles more effectively.

Thomas's life has become quite constricted because almost any location presents potential danger. Needless to say, his wife is quite concerned about his odd beliefs and behaviors and disturbed by their effects on her. She mentions that getting gasoline for the car is left to her because Thomas is unable even to roll down the window in a full-service station. He further involves her in his "habits" by requiring her to wash her hands thoroughly if, while preparing a meal, she touches a doorknob or adjusts the television, thereby "contaminating" her hands.

When Thomas was in his mid-40s, he had experienced a similar episode of fear of particles. The episode had begun when his son-in-law was breaking toothpicks. Thomas thought that a toothpick sliver had flown through the air, fallen into his drink, and subsequently become lodged in his throat. The results of repeated medical examinations were normal, and Thomas received psychiatric treatment (details unknown). Because of or coincidental with treatment, his symptoms remitted after about a year, only to return 20 years later.

DSM-IV Diagnosis

Axis I: 300.3   Obsessive-Compulsive Disorder

Discussion

The longitudinal course of OCD in this patient was unusual. The average age at onset of OCD is late teens to early 20s, with males becoming symptomatic several years earlier than females. Onset after the age of 40 is uncommon; OCD develops in 95% of patients by age 45.[3] The clinical course of OCD can follow several patterns, with the majority of patients (72%) experiencing a chronic waxing and waning course. In 16% of patients, symptoms are continuous, whereas in about 9%, deterioration is progressive. Those patients with a clearly episodic course and periods of complete remission are even less common (about 3%).[4] In earlier writings, considerably higher spontaneous remission rates (25% to 71%) were described. Based on more recent observations, the late onset of the illness and the 20-year symptom-free interval place Thomas in a quite atypical category.

Contamination obsessions usually involve dirt or germs, although toxins, chemicals, cleansers, radiation, and body fluids are sometimes concerns. This patient's fear of particles was somewhat unusual but quite consistent with a contamination obsession, which, in turn, was closely linked to both cleaning and avoidance rituals.

Case Presentation 46
Checking for Tics

Andrew, 68 years of age, has came for evaluation. He retired 3 years earlier from his job as a groundskeeper. He has been married for

---

[3]Black A: "The Natural History of Obsessional Neurosis," in *Obsessional States.* Edited by Beech HR. London, Methuen, 1974, pp. 20–54.

[4]Rasmussen S, Eisen JL: "Phenomenology of OCD: Clinical Subtypes, Heterogeneity and Coexistence," in *The Psychobiology of Obsessive-Compulsive Disorder.* Edited by Zohar J, Insel T, Rasmussen S. New York, Springer, 1991, pp. 13–43.

40 years and has two adult children, who are alive and well. Andrew describes a marriage in which he and his wife have drifted apart, and he thinks that this estrangement is the cause of the depressed mood he has experienced for much of the past 15 years. He is under the care of a local psychiatrist, who has treated him with a monoamine oxidase inhibitor without much benefit. There has never been a full spectrum of neurovegetative symptoms, suicidal ideation, or psychotic symptoms.

When questioned further, Andrew notes that he has always been shy, dating back to childhood. He has felt uncomfortable speaking in public or being under scrutiny, even in small groups. Gradually he reveals that in his 30s he developed the fear that he would make some physical movement or blurt out a word that would be offensive or embarrassing. In fact, although there had been no history of actual tics, Andrew would find himself checking over and over again to make certain that his eyes could track normally from right to left and back again without getting stuck in one position or another. He would also find himself acutely aware of his mouth, checking and rechecking that his lips were not quivering or twitching involuntarily. Not only did these concerns arise when he was in public, but they prevailed as a distraction even when he was alone.

Andrew states that his fears and uncertainty about the movements of his eyes and lips prompted him to avoid going out more than necessary. He managed to function adequately at his job, but since retiring, he has avoided leaving his home except for walks alone or in the company of his dog. This isolation is very upsetting to him because he enjoys the warmth of human connections, such as those he experienced with his former co-workers. He demonstrates substantial insight in that he remains fully aware that his fears are not grounded in reality. This fact further increases his sense of shame.

DSM-IV Diagnoses

Axis I: 300.23   Social Phobia (Social Anxiety Disorder)
           300.3   Obsessive-Compulsive Disorder
           300.4   Dysthymic Disorder

Discussion

Andrew's case highlights the diagnostic difficulty presented by patients with comorbid anxiety disorders, as well as the relationship between OCD and tic disorders.

Andrew had a clear history of symptoms consistent with social phobia. These symptoms included his reliable experience of anxiety when in public, his fear of behaving in a manner that might cause humiliation, and his recognition that his symptoms were excessive. He later developed a pattern of checking behaviors and intrusive thoughts pertaining to his fear of blurting out inappropriate words or sounds. These characteristics are in keeping with a diagnosis of OCD. It is of particular interest that the physical movements about which he became concerned are reminiscent of tics. Indeed, there is a growing body of evidence linking OCD to Tourette's disorder, a disorder that entails both vocal and motor tics (see Case Presentation 40). Andrew does not meet criteria for any tic disorder, never having actually experienced tics. Although his preoccupation is related to a somatic concern, he retains insight and does not meet formal criteria for any somatoform disorder.

Andrew reports chronic dysphoria, and although his case is not fully described, the dysphoria does meet the criteria for dysthymic disorder. It is not uncommon for patients afflicted with OCD and other anxiety disorders to develop secondary mood disturbances. In Andrew's case, he has never satisfied the criteria for a major depressive episode.

Case Presentation 47
Hoarding and the Birth of a Child

Candice is a 26-year-old single mother of a 4-year-old boy. She had an unremarkable early development, although she describes herself as having been a shy child. As an adolescent she rebelled against her parents, culminating in her departure from home shortly after high school graduation. During the years that followed, she led a bohemian lifestyle, working as an artist and pursuing a series of romantic relationships with men with similar interests.

At approximately 19 years of age, Candice entered into a romantic relationship with an artist who was charismatic and overbearing. Gradually she developed some difficulty in discarding items, including old clothing, papers, and trash. She notes that throwing away such items made her feel anxious and depressed. Their apartment became progressively cluttered, but during this period, when pressed, she did manage to discard unneeded objects.

Two years into their relationship, Candice became pregnant. During her pregnancy her boyfriend began spending more and more time away from home and left her permanently before their child was born.

At 22, Candice found herself alone with a newborn son. Subsequently, her hoarding behaviors intensified severely. Specifically, she became entirely unable to throw away anything related to her son. She kept his old clothes, the wrappings from gifts given to him, and even his soiled diapers. She retained insight into the extreme nature of this behavior; nonetheless, she would become intolerably anxious and depressed when she attempted to throw things away. As her apartment grew more and more cluttered, she became increasingly depressed, ultimately exhibiting a full complement of neurovegetative signs.

Treatment with behavior therapy and medication helped with the depression and allowed Candice to limit unsanitary practices. She experienced a major setback, however, when a beloved pet died. She was unable to discard its body and, instead, kept it wrapped in her freezer until, on a home visit, her therapist helped her with its disposal.

Candice remains acutely invested in her child's welfare and deeply ashamed of her hoarding behaviors. Her ability to produce artwork and earn a living has been marginal.

DSM-IV Diagnoses

Axis I: 300.3   Obsessive-Compulsive Disorder
           296.2x   Major Depressive Disorder, Single Episode

Discussion

Candice's case illustrates the primary symptom of hoarding in OCD. This is a controversial issue because hoarding is included under the description of obsessive-compulsive personality disorder (OCPD). Candice's personality style is not in keeping with that of OCPD. Her ritualistic hoarding of objects, the anxiety that she feels when discarding them, her retained insight as to the extreme nature of her behavior, and the gradual decrease in functioning that her symptoms cause all stand as compelling evidence for a diagnosis of OCD.

Although Candice's hoarding symptoms emerged in early adulthood, it is curious that they clearly intensified during the postpartum period. It is not uncommon for OCD symptoms to increase during times of situational stress. The effects of pregnancy on women with OCD have not been formally and prospectively studied. Anecdotally, we have encountered several female patients with OCD whose symptoms emerged or intensified during the postpartum period.

Candice's episode of major depressive disorder appears to be secondary to her OCD. It is common for patients suffering from OCD, especially when the disorder is poorly controlled through treatment, to manifest symptoms of major depression secondarily.

Case Presentation 48
Are They Laughing at Me?

David is a 66-year-old man with a lifelong history of repetitive behaviors. Beginning at approximately 12 years of age, he recalls counting, repeating, ritualized touching, and hand-washing behaviors that, if not performed, led to a feeling of mounting anxiety. Each of the compulsions was performed to neutralize "bad thoughts." These symptoms waxed and waned throughout his childhood and adult life. In spite of them, he earned above-average grades in secondary school, college, and graduate school. He always kept his symptoms hidden, as they were a source of great shame. In his 30s, David married and had a long and successful career as a teacher. He was able to conceal his symptoms from his wife during this time.

In his late 50s, the quality of David's symptoms changed. As he neared retirement age, he began to believe that people at work held him in low regard. Gradually, this feeling generalized to everyone with whom he came in contact, within the workplace and beyond. Although his other compulsive symptoms remained in relatively good control, he developed a complex behavior pattern of questioning persons he met about whether or not they were laughing at him. Of course, the persons whom he encountered in a store or on the street met this question with great surprise. Still, the majority compliantly reassured him that they were not laughing at him. In spite of these reassurances, David felt the need to check by asking the same question of them again and again. His behavior would finally engender amusement or contempt from the bystanders. Sometimes his behavior led to disruptions. On more than one occasion, police were called to the scene because of his persistence. He retained the insight that his behavior was absurd but felt that he could not stop it. At times, the notion that others were laughing at him approached the magnitude of an overvalued idea. Still, David never became delusional.

A comprehensive medical and psychiatric workup did not reveal any evidence of an intercurrent medical cause for these new symptoms. Nor was there any evidence of emergent cognitive dysfunction.

David's symptoms led to his being terminated from his job. Subsequently, a great deal of conflict arose in his marriage because he could no longer conceal his symptoms while remaining at home. An extensive course of behavior therapy allowed him to reestablish a communicative relationship with his wife, but he remains grossly debilitated by his perpetual doubting and quest for reassurance. Exhaustive medication trials have been to no avail.

DSM-IV Diagnosis

Axis I: 300.3   Obsessive-Compulsive Disorder

Discussion

David's case depicts the emergence of new symptoms in a patient with relatively stable OCD for many years.

David's early history is similar to the early history of many OCD patients. His symptoms developed in early adolescence and persisted with a waxing and waning course throughout much of his life. In his late 50s, new symptoms were added to a previously stable set of OCD manifestations. Especially in middle-age and elderly adults, it is imperative to perform a comprehensive workup when such clinical changes occur. In David's case, incipient dementia, primary medical illness, and major depressive disorder were ruled out as impostors of exacerbated OCD. Despite the paranoid flavor of David's new symptoms, there was no evidence that any psychotic process was at work.

It is possible that the exacerbation of David's OCD was attributable to subtle situational stressors surrounding his job or his marriage. It may also be that David's case is simply an example of the unpredictability of the course of OCD.

The following definitions apply:

Obsession: a recurrent intrusive thought recognized as coming from within and as being senseless and irrational (insight preserved).

Overvalued idea: a false belief that is thought to be probably true and that any accompanying rituals are thought to probably negate; represents a transition between an obsession and a delusion.

Delusion: a fixed false belief not recognized as senseless and usually attributed to an outside source (no insight)

CME Test
Chapter 8
Case Presentations 43–48

Please read the six sets of questions (12 questions total) that follow
and circle the one best answer for each question on the corresponding
answer sheet in the accompanying booklet.

Case Presentation 43: The Circumnavigator

43A. Which of the following is *not* an indicator that the patient
has obsessive-compulsive disorder (OCD)?
  1. His turning the car around repeatedly on the way to work
     to be sure he has not struck a pedestrian or caused an
     accident.
  2. His attachment to his mother.
  3. His riding the elevator several times to listen for the phone
     near the elevator door.

43B. Which of the following is an indicator that the patient has
avoidant personality disorder?
  1. He never attends work-related social functions.
  2. He avoids the "sentinel" near the elevator door at work.
  3. His palms became sweaty and he wrung his hands during
     the psychiatric consultation.

Case Presentation 44: His Family's Shame

44A. OCD was an "attractive" diagnosis to the patient's family
because
  1. OCD does not affect the daily life of the patient.
  2. OCD has been relatively well publicized.
  3. The symptoms of OCD are usually more readily treated
     than are those associated with schizophrenia.

44B. OCD is not classified as a psychosis because
  1. No genetic studies have shown linkage between OCD and
     psychoses.

2. Most patients with OCD retain insight into the irrationality of their thoughts and rituals.

3. Rituals of patients with OCD are less bizarre than those of psychotic patients.

Case Presentation 45: The Man Who Feared Particles

45A. The clinical course of OCD
1. Is marked by continuous symptomatology and progressive deterioration in about half of untreated patients.
2. Depends on the patient's sex and his or her age at symptom onset.
3. Can usually be characterized as "waxing and waning."

45B. The fear of "particles" that the patient in this case exhibits
1. Is consistent with a contamination obsession.
2. Came to be shared by his wife, who indulged in his rituals.
3. Has waxed and waned over a 20-year period.

Case Presentation 46: Checking for Tics

46A. The patient's continuous concern that he is exhibiting motor or vocal tics
1. Is characteristic of patients with social phobia.
2. Was exacerbated by his discovery one day that his lips were, in fact, twitching uncontrollably.
3. Is related to both his social phobia and his OCD.

46B. The fact that this patient has dysthymic disorder in addition to OCD and social phobia is
1. Not that surprising, because mood disturbances secondary to anxiety disorders are common.
2. Quite unusual.
3. Probably a coincidence (i.e., due to chance).

Case Presentation 47: Hoarding and the Birth of a Child

47A. Which of the following best distinguishes this patient from a person with obsessive-compulsive personality disorder?
1. Her anxiety when she discards hoarded items.
2. Her shame over her hoarding behavior.
3. Her hoarding behavior.

47B. It is not uncommon for symptoms of OCD to intensify in patients
1. During times of situational stress.
2. During the second trimester in pregnant women.
3. As they age.

Case Presentation 48: Are They Laughing at Me?

48A. A person who has an overvalued idea differs from one with a more characteristic obsession in which of the following respects?
1. He or she recognizes that the notion is irrational.
2. He or she attributes the notion to an external source.
3. He or she believes that the notion may be real.

48B. In this patient's case, which of the following was ruled out as a possible cause of the exacerbation of his OCD?
1. Incipient dementia
2. Marital problems
3. Situational stressors at work

CHAPTER 9

Case Presentation 49
Obsessed With the Departed

An anxiety disorders center was asked by a family physician to evaluate a 78-year-old woman, Dorothy, whose condition had been given a tentative diagnosis of obsessive-compulsive disorder (OCD). Referral information indicated that the patient had been experiencing severe difficulties since the death of her husband, Vernon, 2 years earlier. She had seen her family doctor eight times since Vernon's death. At each appointment she talked incessantly about Vernon, his death, and the need for a "perfect funeral." Although it had been 2 years since her husband died, she was still unable to organize a memorial service. In his will, Vernon had requested that a simple memorial service be held and that his ashes be cast into the ocean near the couple's summer cottage. Trying to respect her deceased husband's wishes, Dorothy had tried on six separate occasions to have a memorial service. Each time she canceled the service because she felt that one detail or another was not satisfactory. The referring physician wondered whether her patient had a variant of OCD exacerbated by the death of her husband.

The patient presented as a sad, elderly appearing woman who was extremely anxious and unable to sit comfortably during the interview. Initially she talked in an extremely rapid monotone about the current plan for Vernon's memorial service. For a time, the psychiatrist allowed her to ramble on about the flower arrangements, music, and eulogy. The discourse was rather disorganized, repetitive, and contradictory. Dorothy's daughter was then asked to join the session to provide her perspective.

141

The daughter explained that her mother actually had had problems before Vernon's sudden and unexpected death. During the months preceding his death, she had become increasingly forgetful and irritable. In fact, Vernon had complained that his wife was up at all hours of the night looking out windows, going through drawers, and wandering aimlessly about the house. Because of these difficulties, he had assumed complete responsibility for management of the family finances, grocery shopping, and other day-to-day activities. After Vernon's death, Dorothy not only had been unable to manage a memorial service but also had allowed unpaid bills and correspondence to accumulate. In addition, she was eating and sleeping sporadically. Her daughter also mentioned that helping her mother was difficult because Dorothy was very suspicious and frequently accused her daughter of trying to steal her money.

As the interview progressed, it became clear that Dorothy had significant cognitive impairment. She was referred to a neurologist, and neuropsychological test results documented a profound cognitive loss. A computed tomography scan demonstrated widened cortical sulci and enlarged ventricles. A diagnosis of dementia of the Alzheimer's type, with late onset and with depressed mood, was made.

DSM-IV Diagnosis

Axis I: 290.21   Dementia of the Alzheimer's Type,
                      With Late Onset, With Depressed Mood

Discussion

Although in OCD and in dementia of the Alzheimer's type, the patient may perseverate excessively on certain topics, the two disorders are readily distinguished by other features. As a rule, patients with OCD have intact cognitive functions, although careful neuropsychological testing may reveal subtle anomalies of visuospatial function that are not usually noticed by the patient or physician. This is in sharp contrast to Alzheimer's dementia, in which impairments are seen in virtually all areas of higher cortical function, such as memory, abstraction, and judgment. In addition, the age at onset for OCD is usually adolescence or early adulthood; onset after age 50 is rare.

Case Presentation 50
The Man Who Couldn't Stop Calling

Recently, an anxiety disorders center was contacted by an attorney requesting an evaluation of one of his clients, Horace, who had been charged with telephone harassment. During the initial telephone call, the lawyer explained that Horace seemed obsessed with his old girlfriend and that this obsession had driven him to commit several illegal acts. The attorney thought that if Horace were suffering from OCD, the diagnosis might be a mitigating factor in the criminal proceedings against him. The attorney explained that over the last several years Horace harassed his ex-girlfriend, Sandy, almost continuously. She had ended her relationship with him years earlier and later married. Yet, Horace was still extremely angry with her.

The police reports forwarded by the attorney described Horace's pattern of harassment. After Sandy ended the relationship, Horace continued to appear unannounced at her home, pounding on her door and demanding to talk. Eventually, Sandy obtained a restraining order that forbade him from coming to her home. This was followed by a relatively quiescent period.

After several months, Sandy reported several acts of minor vandalism to the police. Although Horace was the chief suspect in this property destruction, there was insufficient evidence to bring formal charges against him. He was contacted by the police and again warned to stay away from Sandy's home. At that point Sandy began receiving harassing phone calls. Sandy felt that the calls were being made by Horace; however, the voice was muffled, and it was difficult to be certain who the caller was. Many calls were simply "hang-ups." Again Sandy contacted the police, and they advised her to have the calls traced. Eventually, the calls were traced to a pay phone in Horace's neighborhood, which was staked out by the police. Ultimately, Horace was observed making four calls and was finally arrested in the act of making a harassing phone call. He was charged with a misdemeanor.

At his preliminary hearing, Horace refused to follow the advice of his attorney and demanded a jury trial. His attorney strongly advised him to plead no contest since there was overwhelming evidence that he was guilty. Horace became extremely angry, accused his attorney of having an affair with Sandy, and dismissed him. Later, Horace retained another attorney, who then contacted the anxiety disorders center.

Horace arrived for his appointment very neatly dressed in a business suit. He was abrupt and impatient with the receptionist. During the examination, Horace denied any symptoms of anxiety, mood problems, or psychotic symptoms. He insisted that Sandy was trying to frame him and that he had never done anything illegal in his life. He further insisted that Sandy was at fault and that she had been following him, stealing his mail, and spying on him. When the psychiatrist asked why Sandy would do something like that, Horace replied, "She is trying to get even with me; she would kill me if she could. Now she's even got the police after me. She is very sly. Sandy will do anything to torment me." When asked about the phone calls, Horace stated that he was simply trying to call Sandy to congratulate her on her recent wedding and that she kept hanging up on him. When the examining psychiatrist asked if he could contact Horace's family members to obtain additional information, Horace became angry, stating, "She has got them all on her side too. They will tell you I'm crazy, but that's because she's poisoned their minds with her lies. She has got to be stopped!"

Horace was given the diagnosis of delusional disorder, persecutory type. The psychiatric evaluation was not used in the court proceedings. Horace was convicted, given a sentence of 1-year probation, and fined $500.

DSM-IV Diagnosis

Axis I: 297.1   Delusional Disorder, Persecutory Type

Discussion

Like OCD, delusional disorder involves chronic recurrent thoughts with an obsessional quality. However, in delusional disorder these thoughts usually have a paranoid or grandiose theme, which is rarely the case with OCD. Also, OCD is usually associated with the patient's recognition of the senselessness of his or her symptoms, whereas delusional disorder is characterized by a lack of insight. Finally, although patients with delusional disorder (persecutory type) commonly avoid certain people or situations, they do not exhibit such compulsive behaviors as hand-washing or dressing rituals, which are typically seen in patients with OCD.

The definitions of an obsession, an overvalued idea, and a delusion provided in the discussion of Case Presentation 48 apply here.

Case Presentation 51
The Law-and-Order Student

Walter, age 25, comes well prepared to his psychiatric evaluation. A slender, reserved, carefully dressed young man, Walter seems keen on being in control: he is organized, poised, and pleasant, and he narrates his difficulties with objective precision. Walter is also remarkably lacking in emotional expression, speaking even of his relationship with his recent girlfriend in words of possession rather than affection. Walter knows he has OCD; in fact, he has apparently read so much about the disorder that it makes the interviewer feel a bit nervous.

Walter says that he has had OCD since high school but that it has worsened since he started law school 2 years ago. Even when sitting in class, he is constantly preoccupied with intrusive thoughts: Is the lighting in the room sufficient? Am I sitting properly, or am I ruining my back? Is this a good pen? Is this desk sufficiently stable? He is constantly worried about causing harm to himself by catching the flu, tripping on a crack between the tiles, or falling off a treacherous chair. He also thinks he might inadvertently hurt others who might catch something from him, or that they might slip on a puddle he has created with his dripping umbrella. Therefore, he checks the safety of electric switches, the strength of furniture, and the hazards of cracks and water puddles on the sidewalk. Walter has mental rituals as well. When furniture looks unsafe, he takes it apart and puts it together again in his mind's eye; when obsessions of harm invade his consciousness, he balances them with corrective counterthoughts. Walter also has had a long-standing fear of receiving injections, which cause him to faint, and he has avoided even necessary medical treatments for that reason.

Walter's parents are Holocaust survivors, and he is their youngest son, having lived alone with them since the age of 11. He has always been driven to do his very best, determined to go further in life than his simple, lower–social class parents, perhaps carrying their ambitions as well as his own. He has been remarkably successful in this mission, despite his OCD, excelling in high school and so far surviving the demands of law school. On the other hand, his social life has always been meager and a source of dissatisfaction, even despair. He reports that he feels rejected by his peers and has never been able to find even a single dependable, intimate friend. Until recently, he had never had what he could term a girlfriend, though there had been isolated sexual contacts. Walter seems quite unsure about his new relationship and is worried that his girlfriend might leave him at any time.

Walter's life has followed a predictable, tightly defined routine; surprises bother him. Walter plans everything to the last detail and is very organized, scheduling his time and arranging his belongings by well-defined criteria. He describes himself as a perfectionist, one who compulsively writes and rewrites every school assignment, with the result that he is barely able to finish on time. He has great difficulty simply relaxing and enjoying himself; he always feels driven, intense, and task oriented. At the same time, simple decisions are excruciatingly difficult to make. He must list the "fors" and "againsts," and he becomes obsessed with each option. He can never quite make up his mind. He is bound to regret and reconsider whatever decision he reaches.

DSM-IV Diagnoses

Axis I: 300.3   Obsessive-Compulsive Disorder
           300.29   Specific Phobia, Blood-Injection-Injury Type
Axis II: 301.4   Obsessive-Compulsive Personality Disorder

Discussion

Walter clearly meets the criteria for OCD with his multiple obsessions and both behavioral and mental rituals. He also meets the criteria for blood-injection-injury phobia, which results in his avoiding medical procedures. But his lifelong pattern of perfectionism, rigid routine, and impoverished interpersonal relationships suggests, in addition, the existence of a personality disorder. Specifically, Walter's perfectionism, preoccupation with order, excessive devotion to work, indecisiveness, and restricted expression of affection are sufficient for the diagnosis of obsessive-compulsive personality disorder (OCPD).

Much has been said already in this casebook about the similarities and differences between OCD and OCPD. These two disorders were traditionally seen by psychoanalytic theorists as reflecting the same unconscious conflicts and defenses, varying only by degree of adaptivity. The descriptive approach taken by the DSM-III-R has not been in accord with this theoretical view, and no clear or necessary relationship between the two disorders is assumed today. In fact, modern studies using DSM-III-R diagnostic criteria have found limited comorbidity between the two disorders.[1] In one study, when the Structured Interview for the DSM-III Personality Disorders (SIDP) was used, only 6% of patients with OCD also met the criteria for OCPD. When the broader criteria in DSM-III-R were applied, 25% of 59 patients with OCD were diagnosed as also having OCPD.

---

[1]Baer L, Jenike MA, Ricciardi JN, et al.: "Standardized Assessment of Personality Disorders in OCD." *Archives of General Psychiatry* 47:826–830, 1990.

Case Presentation 52
Obsessed With Hunger

Ted is a 26-year-old man who recalls mild OCD symptoms beginning at approximately 10 years of age. These symptoms included touching walls and counting to neutralize anxiety associated with thoughts that if he did not perform these rituals, "something bad would happen." Despite these symptoms, he was able to continue his school activities. The rituals became much less prominent after Ted was about 13 years of age, although some waxing and waning were observed. At presentation, Ted reported preoccupation with symmetry and with the arrangements of objects on desks and walls. He also turned doorknobs in certain ways before opening doors and touched objects a specific number of times and in a predetermined order. These symptoms caused only minor impairment. In high school, Ted became more preoccupied than most teenagers with aspects of his physical appearance, including his weight. Gradually he focused single-mindedly on becoming thin. Still, he never severely restricted dietary intake, exercised to excess, abused laxatives or diuretics, or made himself vomit. He denies any history of bingeing. He was never obese nor less than 85% of the ideal body weight for his height and age. In spite of his preoccupation with weight, there was no evidence that Ted had a grossly distorted body image or a misperception that he was disfigured in any way.

Ted was a successful high school athlete and earned mostly A's in his classes. Although orderly and well organized, he was neither rigid in his daily activities nor perfectionistic in his personality style. In college, he continued his preoccupation with thinness while earning average grades. After Ted was graduated from college, his focus on thinness intensified and he began to read voraciously about nutrition, diets, and control of eating behaviors.

Two years before presentation, Ted began to abuse nonprescription diet pills (phenylpropanolamine), which allowed him to control his appetite and lose small amounts of weight. He used up to 10 times the recommended dose of these medications for 6 months before stopping abruptly when he became convinced that this practice was medically unwise. Upon discontinuing the medication he developed an overwhelming physical sensation of hunger, perhaps initially reflecting a rebound phenomenon. This hunger, which he described as unyielding and insatiable, has persisted to the present.

Ted's hunger interfered with his concentration and frequently awakened him from sleep. He was extensively evaluated medically, but no organic cause of his symptoms was found. Thinking incessantly of food, he went from specialist to specialist in search of an explanation for his condition. Trials of a variety of psychiatric medications were to no avail. He expressed the insight that he was obsessed both with thinness and with the cause of his hunger. Subsequently, Ted became somewhat depressed, but he has no history of psychosis, mania, suicidal ideation, or panic attacks.

DSM-IV Diagnoses

Axis I: 300.3   Obsessive-Compulsive Disorder
          307.50   Eating Disorder Not Otherwise Specified
          305.70   Amphetamine Abuse

Discussion

Ted's case raises a difficult question about the relationship between OCD and eating disorders.

Certainly, patients presenting with characteristic features of eating disorders routinely have unwanted thoughts and repetitive ritualized behaviors as part of their illness. Although DSM-III-R specifically stated that these symptoms cannot be accepted as meeting the criteria for OCD, DSM-IV permits diagnosis of OCD in the presence of another Axis I disorder as long as "the content of the obsessions or compulsions is not restricted to it."[2] Ted's case is unique in two ways. First, there is a known history of hallmark OCD symptoms. Second, Ted's preoccupation with thinness does not follow the typical pattern of either anorexia nervosa or bulimia

---

[2]American Psychiatric Association: *Diagnostic and Statistical Manual of Mental Disorders*, 4th Edition. Washington, D.C., American Psychiatric Association, 1994, p. 423.

nervosa. Also, his self-concept is not distorted in the manner required for a diagnosis of body dysmorphic disorder. It is not unreasonable to suspect that there may be a relationship between Ted's OCD and the development of his coexisting eating disorder and that his hunger may be the result of a truly obsessional preoccupation. Alternatively, Ted's eating disorder may reflect changes secondary to chronic appetite suppression.

Ted's abuse of sympathomimetic "diet pills" is an important component of his history as well. Although his OCD symptoms had emerged previously, there is some suggestion that his use or discontinuation of the medication may have contributed to the exacerbation of OCD symptoms. Results in the literature on the influence of psychostimulants on OCD symptoms are mixed. Induction,[3] exacerbation,[4] and attenuation[5] of OCD symptoms in response to psychostimulant use have all been reported.

Case Presentation 53
He Sinned in His Heart

Charles, a 43-year-old married auto mechanic and father of two daughters, seeks psychiatric treatment, complaining of mood swings with a tendency to remain depressed. He confides, "I was so low

[3] Borcherding BG, Keysor CS, Rapoport JL, et al.: "Motor/Vocal Tics and Compulsive Behaviors on Stimulant Drugs: Is There a Common Vulnerability?" *Psychiatry Research* 33:83–94, 1990; Satel SL, McDougle CJ: "Obsessions and Compulsions Associated With Cocaine Abuse (Letter)." *American Journal of Psychiatry* 148:947, 1991.

[4] McDougle CJ, Goodman WK, Delgado PL, et al.: "Pathophysiology of Obsessive-Compulsive Disorder (Letter)." *American Journal of Psychiatry* 146:1350–1351, 1989.

[5] Joffe RT, Swinson RP, Levitt AJ: "Acute Psychostimulant Challenge in Primary Obsessive-Compulsive Disorder." *Journal of Clinical Psychopharmacology* 11:237–241, 1991.

yesterday, I felt I could no longer continue to live."

Charles reveals that he is running out of things to tell his wife, things that he did wrong to her and to others throughout his life. "Five years ago, while I was driving, bang, a thought hit my mind that I had cheated on my wife 10 years earlier. A year later I told her about it . . . and since then I have been thinking about it over and over again." The extent of his marital infidelity was that many times he put his wife "in second place" in his thoughts. In other words, he thought about other women, too, although he had never actually had any physical contact with them. "Now, I have to tell my wife everything I have done over the past ?? years." All the Mickey Mouse stuff . . . I know it's ridiculous, but I have to tell her everything. She's sick of it, and I am too!"

Charles reports that for the past 16 years he has been in psychotherapy because of his "personality problems." He says that for many years he was completely unable to stand it if anyone disliked him—that he could not forget and would be "consumed with it" to the point of depression. As he describes the problem, "I am fixated on people. If they like me, I am happy. But if they don't, I am very miserable. I can't let go of it. I have to think about what they dislike about me over and over again. When I run out of things they dislike, I start to think about what I have done wrong to myself and my wife."

With the help of a Christian counselor, Charles felt that he had overcome his "fixation on people" when he became a born-again Christian 11 years ago. He still believes that he has repented but questions, "Why am I still feeling guilty? Didn't I really repent?" Without any known stressors, he has obsessed for the past 5 years about having done something wrong to others. "Doc, I'm out of control. I cannot stop saying something that I am guilty of." His latest preoccupation is that he is "morally depraved" because recently, as he entered his family bathroom with a clean towel for his 10-year-old daughter, he saw her naked body through the frosted glass door of the shower stall. His confession of this event to his wife has caused him great pain and has left him very depressed.

Charles reveals that when he was newly married, at age 21, he bought his first car, which he had to check more than 10 times every night to be sure he had locked all the doors and turned off the lights.

His wife thought his behavior was peculiar but made little of it because it lasted only a few weeks and never recurred. Four years later his pattern of fixation on people began and continued for approximately 7 years. The present confessional period developed 5 years ago and has been ongoing.

DSM-IV Diagnoses

Axis I: 300.3   Obsessive-Compulsive Disorder
Axis II: 301.6   Dependent Personality Disorder

Discussion

The possibility that Charles is suffering from a primary depressive disorder has been ruled out because his depressive state is secondary to his obsessive ruminations and compulsive confessions. Although his depressive symptoms are fairly intense, there are no concomitant depressive neurovegetative symptoms and signs. He does not suffer from fatigue or lack of motivation, and despite the "mood swings" he initially reported, there has been no true cyclothymic or hypomanic episode.

The "personality problems" Charles describes are, viewed retrospectively, largely the manifestations of OCD with onset in early adulthood and a waxing and waning of symptoms during the last several years. His symptoms are senseless to him, and he knows that they are the product of his own mind, not imposed on his mind from external sources. This latter feature makes it easy to rule out any delusional disorders or morbid religious fanaticism and points to a diagnosis of OCD.

Although Charles is overly conscientious and scrupulous in his thoughts, he lacks other obsessive-compulsive personality characteristics such as perfectionism, indecisiveness, and morbid preoccupation with details, rules, or organization. Instead, he is easily hurt by others' dislikes, criticism, or disapproval and is dependent on his wife's reassurance and "absolution" in the wake of his guilt-ridden reports. This latter feature points to a diagnosis of dependent personality disorder rather than obsessive-compulsive personality disorder. Dependent personality disorder is often associated with OCD and, in fact, may sometimes be secondary to OCD, as evidenced by improvement in the personality disorder when the OCD is effectively treated.[6]

Case Presentation 54
Stuck on His Tics

Jerry is a 25-year-old waiter who complains that his "mind keeps getting stuck" and that it is "driving [him] nuts." Sometimes he feels only death will grant him relief. Once a disturbing thought enters his mind, it lingers until he successfully performs a neutralizing behavior. His parents have insisted that he see a psychiatrist.

The majority of Jerry's recurring thoughts concern whether he has done things correctly or carefully enough. He fears that he may be responsible for something going wrong that will cost him his job or jeopardize the welfare of others. At work, Jerry's boss has reproached him for being late to work and for being so inefficient. After taking an order, he begins to doubt whether he got it right, and often has to go back to the customer and review which menu items were selected. Before leaving the house, Jerry repeatedly checks that the stove is off, the faucets are shut off, and the door is locked. This can take more than an hour.

Jerry also describes a variety of nearly irresistible urges that occur in the absence of antecedent thoughts or fears. For example, he may spontaneously experience a need to touch, tap, or rub objects. He sometimes spends hours rearranging and aligning objects such as stationery supplies; if something is moved as little as one millimeter, the whole process may have to be repeated. The height of his socks and the tension in his shoelaces have to be adjusted until "it feels just right."

---

[6]Baer L, Jenike MA, Black DW, et al.: "Effect of Axis II Diagnoses on Treatment Outcome With Clomipramine in 55 Patients With Obsessive-Compulsive Disorder." *Archives of General Psychiatry* 49:862–866, 1992.

Although he denies any recent stressors, it is clear that Jerry is feeling pressure to earn enough money to move out of his parents' house. He had been hoping for a promotion but now fears losing his job. For the last 3 weeks he has been experiencing increased hopelessness about his future. Jerry thinks about committing suicide, but his religious convictions make this act untenable. Although he reports feeling depressed, Jerry still enjoys going bowling, looks forward to seeing his girlfriend, and displays a full range of affect. He reports difficulty falling asleep but denies other neurovegetative signs or symptoms of depression.

Jerry reports that he first felt there was something wrong shortly after his eighth birthday. At that time, his classmates started to make fun of his body movements, which included bouts of forceful eye blinking, shoulder shrugging, and neck jerking. His parents referred to these as "bad habits" that he should work harder to control. Two years later, in addition to motor tics, he developed repetitive throat clearing, sniffing, and barking sounds that brought him to the attention of his pediatrician. A neurologist was consulted and made the diagnosis of Tourette's disorder.

DSM-IV Diagnoses

Axis I: 300.3   Obsessive-Compulsive Disorder
            307.23   Tourette's Disorder
Axis II: 799.9   Diagnosis Deferred

Discussion

The patient reports recurrent and disturbing thoughts that he experiences as intrusive, as well as a need to perform behaviors that seem designed to counteract the discomfort triggered by these thoughts. Jerry's obsessions and compulsions involve content and form typical of patients with OCD. His principal obsessions concern themes of safety and harm and a need for exactness, and his compulsions include checking and repeating behaviors. That these symptoms are interfering with his vocational functioning and occupy more than an hour each day clearly qualifies him for a diagnosis of OCD.

In addition, Jerry has had a diagnosis of Tourette's disorder since age 8. Criteria for Tourette's disorder include onset before age 21 and chronic multiple motor tics and one or more vocal tics. Tourette's disorder is three to five times more common in males than in females. Obsessive-compulsive symptoms occur in approximately 50% of patients with Tourette's disorder and may not appear until late childhood or early adulthood (see Case Presentation 40). As in Jerry's case, obsessions and compulsions may replace the tics as the dominant clinical problem. It is not clear whether Jerry's need to touch, tap, and rub objects is best classified as involving complex motor tics or compulsions

The patient complains of depressed mood, insomnia, and suicidal ideation for a period of more than 2 weeks. However, he does not qualify for a DSM-IV diagnosis of major depressive disorder, which requires the presence of at least two more symptoms. Nevertheless, he should be monitored carefully for the development of a full depressive episode.

Diagnosis of a Axis II disorder(s) was properly deferred because the clinician did not have enough information and experience with Jerry to form an accurate opinion about disorders on this axis.

CME Test
Chapter 9
Case Presentations 49–54

Please read the six sets of questions (12 questions total) that follow and circle the one best answer for each question on the corresponding answer sheet in the accompanying booklet.

Case Presentation 49: Obsessed With the Departed

49A. Which of the following factors does *not* reliably differentiate obsessive-compulsive disorder (OCD) from dementia of the Alzheimer's type?
1. Age at onset of symptoms.
2. Degree of loss of cognitive function.
3. Presence (or absence) of perseveration.

49B. Which of the following would most strongly suggest the preliminary tentative diagnosis of OCD made in this case?
1. The rapid, monotonous, and disorganized nature of the patient's monologue about her husband's memorial service.
2. The fact that the patient had canceled six memorial services because she felt that one detail or another was not satisfactory.
3. The fact that the patient's daughter revealed that the patient had actually had problems *before* her husband's death.

Case Presentation 50: The Man Who Couldn't Stop Calling

50A. Although he has delusional disorder, the patient exhibits what symptom characteristic of persons with OCD?
1. Recurrent thoughts with an obsessional quality.
2. Insight into the senselessness of his actions.
3. Unusually tidy dress.

50B. The obsessive thoughts of a person with delusional disorder
1. Are transient in nature.

2. Are often exacerbated by the person's frustration at being aware they are irrational.
3. Can usually be characterized as paranoid or grandiose.

Case Presentation 51: The Law-and-Order Student

51A. Which does *not* apply to patients with obsessive-compulsive personality disorder (OCPD)?
1. They tend to be perfectionistic.
2. They may find decision making excruciatingly difficult.
3. In most cases OCD is a comorbid condition.

51B. Which of the following symptoms exhibited by Walter does *not* suggest OCPD?
1. His lack of emotional expression.
2. His fear of injections.
3. His task-oriented behavior.

Case Presentation 52: Obsessed With Hunger

52A. Which of the following is true of this patient's insatiable hunger?
1. It was relieved by psychiatric medications.
2. It could be the result of an obsession and thus related to his OCD.
3. It suggests that he suffers from bulimia.

52B. The patient's abuse of diet pills may have contributed to
1. His symptoms of anorexia nervosa.
2. His grossly distorted body image.
3. The exacerbation of his OCD symptoms.

Case Presentation 53: He Sinned in His Heart

53A. The present depressed mood of this patient
1. Alternates with periods of euphoric relief at having "come clean."
2. Is a product of his continual guilt-ridden ruminations and confessions.
3. Is accompanied by a paralyzing lack of motivation.

53B. In dependent personality disorder comorbid with OCD
   1. Successful treatment of the OCD may demonstrate that the dependent personality disorder was secondary to the OCD.
   2. OCPD would be a third likely comorbid condition.
   3. The dependent personality disorder is unlikely to improve with successful treatment of the OCD.

Case Presentation 54: Stuck on His Tics

54A. According to this case presentation, what percentage of persons who suffer from Tourette's disorder also have OCD?
   1. 40% to 60%.
   2. The case discussion refers to obsessive-compulsive symptoms, not the full-criteria disorder.
   3. 5% to 10%.

54B. The patient's spontaneous touching, tapping, and rubbing of objects represent
   1. Complex motor tics.
   2. Compulsions.
   3. Either tics or compulsions.

Case Presentation 55
The Boy Who Would Not Behave

Jamie, a 12-year-old boy, was referred by his school psychologist because he was refusing to attend school. Before the appointment his school records were forwarded, along with a psychological evaluation done by the referring psychologist. The records indicated that Jamie had missed nearly 100 days of school during the current school year and a similar number during the previous year.

Because of conduct problems, Jamie had been placed in foster care about 8 months ago. His foster parents described him as a quiet, secretive boy who frequently refused to come out of his room. When his foster parents attempted to force him to get ready for school, he would become extremely angry and verbally abusive. The psychologist's evaluation indicated that Jamie had depressive symptoms and low self-esteem, and his condition was diagnosed as oppositional defiant disorder. The referring psychologist had requested further evaluation because the situation was approaching a crisis. Jamie had not been in school for 2 weeks and almost never came out of his room, and the foster parents were considering having him removed from their home.

Jamie was 45 minutes late for the interview and arrived in an irritable, sullen mood. His foster parents reported that it was extremely difficult to get him out of his room and into the car to come for the appointment. During the initial part of the interview, his foster parents described at length how exasperated they were with his slowness. They had tried nagging, rewarding, and punishing, all to no avail. Furthermore, when they attempted to hurry Jamie, he would become enraged and scream obscenities at them. When Jamie was asked what was behind these difficulties, he simply shrugged his shoulders and said, "I don't know."

The second half of the interview was conducted with Jamie alone. Because of his angry and upset mood, the interview initially focused on a neutral subject: his favorite popular music band. Jamie soon relaxed, talked in an animated manner, and did not appear at all depressed. During the course of the interview, Jamie admitted that he actually enjoyed school and that he regretted missing so many classes. When asked why it was so difficult for him to get to school, he replied in a halting voice, "It's really stupid, but I just have to do certain things." With much encouragement Jamie was able to confide that he had a terrifying feeling that something dreadful would happen if he did not dress himself, brush his teeth, and do other things in groups of four. If any of these rituals was not performed correctly, Jamie felt that he had to go back to the very beginning and repeat them all four times. Thus, when his foster parents tried to hurry him along, he soon became frustrated and angry.

DSM-IV Diagnosis

Axis I: 300.3   Obsessive-Compulsive Disorder

Discussion

Like many other children with obsessive-compulsive disorder (OCD), Jamie became very upset when his rituals were interrupted. He was too embarrassed by the senseless nature of his obsessional thoughts and compulsive activities to confide in his foster parents. Believing that Jamie was simply being difficult and disobedient, they felt it important to enforce strict discipline, worsening the situation. Fortunately, correct identification of the nature of Jamie's difficulties enabled him to receive appropriate treatment instead of being placed in another foster home.

Many children (and adults) are so ashamed of their OCD symptoms that they keep them secret for years. Children and adolescents are reluctant to tell their therapists about OCD symptoms, and their omission of these details can result in the wrong diagnosis. In Jamie's case, it is possible that unrecognized OCD caused the conduct problems that led to the foster care placement and to the diagnosis of oppositional defiant disorder.

Although OCD is an unusual cause of behavioral problems in children, the presence of this disorder should always be considered, especially when the behavior problems are associated with seemingly minor interruptions in the child's day-to-day activities.

Case Presentation 56
Obsessed With Her Fears

Jennifer is a 28-year-old, single woman who is employed as a bank manager. At the time she is initially evaluated, she is living alone. Jennifer is obsessed with intrusive and graphic images of being the victim of a violent crime. For 2 years before she sought psychiatric attention, Jennifer would spend several hours each evening checking to make certain that her doors and windows were locked and secure. She also would spend a good deal of each evening checking the street outside her house to make certain no strangers were parked there. Jennifer had replaced the locks on her doors several times in the past 6 months because of fears that they were malfunctioning or worries that she had left her key where it could have been copied during the day. Although Jennifer had initially been satisfied to check her locks once, she had gradually become ever more doubtful that she had really made things secure. The week of the evaluation, Jennifer reported that she was checking the door about 50 times per night. Her sleep was severely disrupted because on awakening during the middle of the night she again felt compelled to go through her checking routine.

During the months leading up to the evaluation, Jennifer had become less successful in her attempts to divert her thoughts. In fact, the more she tried to put them out of her mind, the more intrusive and frequent the images became. Jennifer also noted new urges to check other "threats," including electrical appliances, water faucets, and household cleansers.

Although Jennifer is capable of working, she has become increasingly wary and concerned about being attacked going to and from her job. She avoids corners where she would have to stop at stoplights and has begun checking the locks on her car. Because of her fears, she has eliminated all social contacts except for those with her immediate family and has refused numerous dates at her office. Although Jennifer is a very attractive woman, she had not gone out with anyone during the 2 years before the evaluation.

Jennifer had been shy and behaviorally inhibited as a child. She had multiple fears and phobias that have persisted since childhood but have never really interfered with her functioning. Both her mother and sister are described as worriers, and her mother has a probable history of panic attacks with a brief period of agoraphobia. Jennifer had never sought psychiatric care before responding to a newspaper article describing OCD and the treatments available at the clinic. On further reflection she remembers having washed her hands excessively, but she reported that this behavior had ceased by the time she was 12 years of age. A careful evaluation elicits no evidence of physical or sexual abuse. Jennifer does report that her fear had greatly intensified 2 years before, after she had seen a movie about a deranged killer.

In addition to her intrusive thoughts, images, and compulsions, Jennifer has many other anxiety-related symptoms. During the past 6 months she experienced several full-blown panic attacks each month. Although they had initially been related to her fear of attack, some appeared to come "out of the blue." On several occasions, Jennifer wakened from sleep with panic symptoms, which were often precipitated by nightmares that she could remember in vivid detail. Symptoms of major depressive disorder were also present over at least 3 months. She reports depressed mood, anhedonia, difficulty concentrating, feelings of hopelessness, insomnia with trouble falling asleep, and early-morning awakening. She had lost 10 pounds over the 2 months before the evaluation. There is no history of depressive disorder, nor is there a positive family history for depression.

On mental status examination Jennifer exhibits a great deal of psychomotor agitation. She is hypervigilant, frequently wrings her hands, and exhibits a markedly potentiated startle response to an unexpected stimulus. She complains of numerous somatic symptoms consistent with sympathetic hyperactivity. In addition, she reports panic attacks, obsessions and compulsions, and symptoms of generalized anxiety. She is moderately depressed and has no suicidal ideation. There are no cognitive deficits. The results of a physical examination and routine laboratory tests are within normal limits.

DSM-IV Diagnoses

Axis I: 300.3   Obsessive-Compulsive Disorder
          296.22 Major Depressive Disorder, Single Episode, Moderate
          300.01 Panic Disorder Without Agoraphobia

Discussion

Jennifer's presentation and history illustrate the extensive comorbidity with other psychiatric conditions characteristic of OCD. Major depressive disorder is the most frequently identified comorbid disorder; 67% of patients with OCD in one large series had experienced at least one episode during their lifetime, and 31% were reported as currently meeting the criteria for major depressive disorder.[1] Often, as in this case, the depressive symptoms are secondary to OCD,[2] and effective treatment of OCD may lead to their resolution as well.

Most of Jennifer's panic attacks were triggered by her obsessional fears, but she did experience unexpected (i.e., uncued) panic attacks that were distressing and warrant a diagnosis of panic disorder without agoraphobia. Similarly, Jennifer's phobic symptoms do not interfere with her functioning sufficiently enough to warrant a formal diagnosis. Panic disorder and both specific and social phobias are, however, prevalent in patients with OCD. In the series referred to previously, 12% of patients with OCD had current or previous panic disorder, 22% had specific phobia, and 18% had

---

[1]Rasmussen SA, Eisen JL: "Clinical Features and Phenomenology of Obsessive Compulsive Disorder." *Psychiatric Annals* 19:67–73, 1989.

[2]Op. cit.

social phobia.[3] Complaints of generalized anxiety, such as Jennifer's, are also common among patients with OCD.[4]

Jennifer's OCD symptoms include avoidance, which is sometimes overlooked as a ritualistic behavior. Her avoidance should be properly considered a compulsion because, like her checking, it is repetitive and purposeful, performed to neutralize the anxiety resulting from obsessive thoughts, and recognized by the patient to be excessive.

For several reasons, Jennifer's avoidant behaviors fail to satisfy the criteria for avoidant personality disorder. Jennifer lacks the pervasive impairment of personal interactions characteristic of avoidant personality disorder. Her avoidant behaviors developed acutely, rather than in the chronic, lifelong course typical of patients with avoidant personality disorder. Moreover, Jennifer's behaviors were clearly related to her obsessional fears and abated as her OCD responded to treatment. Personality disorders are expected to be lifelong and persist despite effective treatment of Axis I disorders.

A diagnosis of delusional (paranoid) disorder, persecutory type, was considered but rejected because Jennifer never believed that a particular person or persons were seeking to harm her, nor was she convinced that something in particular was going to happen. Rather, her fears grew out of a general sense that something terrible could happen. Again, her fears were clearly related to her obsessions and largely resolved in response to treatment.

Case Presentation 57
The Boy Who Collected Soda Cans

Nicholas, a 10-year-old, is referred for evaluation because of difficulty making friends at school. According to his mother, Nicholas

---

[3] Rasmussen SA, Eisen JL: "Clinical Features and Phenomenology of Obsessive Compulsive Disorder." *Psychiatric Annals* 19:67–73, 1989.

[4] Rasmussen SA, Eisen JL: "Clinical Features and Phenomenology of Obsessive Compulsive Disorder." *Psychiatric Annals* 19:67–73, 1989; Pitman RK, Green RC, Jenike MA, et al.: "Clinical Comparison of Tourette's Disorder and OCD." *American Journal of Psychiatry* 144:1166–1171, 1987.

has always been extremely shy. She is concerned because her son seems fascinated with collecting soda cans. He takes any soda can he finds to his room and keeps it there. There are piles of cans in his room, and he refuses to allow any of them to be thrown out.

Nicholas also seems uninterested in forming friendships at school and has difficulty with the basic skills involved in making friends. He interacts with peers only if they participate in collecting cans with him. Nicholas never participates in play acting and shows no interest in stories about imaginary events. He shows some delay in speech and often repeats the last phrase used by others around him. When he speaks, his words tend to be very high pitched and abnormal in rhythm. Unable to keep conversations going with his peers, Nicholas tends to become silent. He has difficulty whenever the routine at home is changed. Occasionally he plays a game with another child, but it has to follow exactly the same rules and routine every time.

When asked about his interest in soda cans, Nicholas cannot explain it but says that collecting cans is fun and that he just has to collect them. He also cannot explain why none of the cans may be thrown out. He does nothing with his cans except look at them. Nicholas spends 2 to 3 hours per day with his cans. Whenever he is out walking, he feels that he must look for soda cans to take home for his collection. On one occasion, Nicholas elected to go to a park with his parents to look for soda cans rather than go to a friend's birthday party.

Nicholas received drug therapy for OCD and showed marked improvement, but only with regard to his collecting of soda cans. He can now go to the park with his parents without looking for cans, but Nicholas's social skills remain extremely poor. Behavioral approaches to treating his pervasive developmental disorder have been unsuccessful. Parental education and the establishment of more realistic social goals have allowed Nicholas's mother to accept her son's underlying condition and to adjust his environment so that he is not pressured excessively.

DSM-IV Diagnoses

Axis I: 300.3   Obsessive-Compulsive Disorder
Axis II: 299.80   Pervasive Developmental Disorder
                      Not Otherwise Specified

Discussion

The case of this 10-year-old boy provides a clear illustration of the recurrent and persistent ideas and impulses that, even to him, appear senseless. It is clear that Nicholas's compulsive collecting of soda cans is time-consuming and interferes significantly with his routine and social functioning. The obsessive-compulsive features of Nicholas's disorder were somewhat hidden by a very prominent pervasive developmental disorder. Some overlap is evident in that pervasive developmental disorders are often characterized by a restricted repertoire of activities and interests, which are frequently stereotyped and repetitive, and by some impairment in communication and social interaction. The stereotypies associated with these disorders, however, can often be distinguished from true compulsive rituals by the patient's absence of insight into their excessive or unreasonable nature.

Case Presentation 58
The Roots of Her Problems

For the past 2 months, it has been obvious to Allison's parents that their daughter has been pulling out her hair. Allison, a girl almost 12 years of age, has thick, long hair on the sides of her head but very sparse, short, broken hairs on her forehead and crown, as well as several areas that are almost devoid of hair. Allison tried to hide this behavior from her parents, but teachers advised them to seek help.

Allison's parents consulted a dermatologist and a psychologist, but Allison continued to pull out large amounts of hair. In desperation, they requested psychiatric evaluation. Allison's parents also described personality changes. Allison had begun to talk incessantly, refusing to be interrupted. In school, she spoke constantly about her 6-month-old brother, Eric. Her peers had begun to avoid her, which caused Allison to cry and feel rejected. She became excessively concerned about minor physical problems and went to the school nurse's office frequently. She also began to check her work repeatedly to the point that she could no longer complete all her assignments.

On evaluation, Allison stated that she feels compelled to pull out her hair so that she can examine the roots. Allison claimed that this does not hurt and that she feels better when she looks at the roots. Allison was wearing a hair band in an attempt to cover her scalp, but the patchy, bald areas were obvious. Her scalp appeared normal, without scarring or signs of inflammation. Allison used to pull out her eyelashes as well but does not mutilate herself in any other way. Although she feels rejected by her peers, she denies feelings of depression.

Allison's mother has been depressed since Eric was born. She also reported an exacerbation of her many compulsions and fears, which include hand washing, house cleaning, fears of various household chemicals, and avoidance of certain areas of carpeting in her home. Her husband has been tolerant of this behavior, but she recognizes that she has forced him to comply with her compulsions and that his frustration tolerance for her symptoms is at its limit.

DSM-IV Diagnoses

Axis I: 312.39   Trichotillomania
            300.3   Obsessive-Compulsive Disorder

Discussion

Allison's symptoms plainly meet DSM-IV criteria for trichotillomania. Upon further review, it is apparent that her symptoms also satisfy the criteria for OCD. In this case, the patient describes an obsession to see her hair roots, resulting in hair pulling. Her earlier incessant chatter about her baby brother also had a compulsive aspect. Allison's excessive concern about her health and schoolwork had led to her compulsive checking with the nurse and of her work.

Allison's mother, likewise, has OCD. Given the timing of the onset of Allison's symptoms, it is reasonable to interpret them as a request for reassurance from a child stressed by the birth of a brother, her mother's disorder, and possible friction between her parents.

Although classified as an impulse-control disorder, along with kleptomania, pyromania, pathological gambling, and intermittent explosive disorder, trichotillomania is often referred to as an "OCD spectrum disorder." There are intriguing similarities between trichotillomania and OCD.[5] Hair pulling is often described as a habit or compulsion that is ego-dystonic, unreasonable, and frequently resisted. However, repetitive rituals in OCD have the seeming purpose of neutralizing anxiety by preventing or producing some future event, which is not the case in trichotillomania. Whereas OCD is thoroughly ego-dystonic, some patients describe a pleasurable or tension-releasing effect to hair pulling. Patients with trichotillomania only rarely have other concomitant OCD symptoms such as washing or checking rituals.[6] OCD is equally common in males and females (but more common in boys than in girls during childhood), but most patients with trichotillomania are women, with onset usually noted during childhood.[7] And, studies using positron-

[5]Hollander E: "Serotonergic Drugs and the Treatment of Disorders Related to Obsessive-Compulsive Disorder," in *Current Treatments of Obsessive-Compulsive Disorder.* Edited by Pato MT, Zohar J. Washington, D.C., American Psychiatric Press, 1991, pp. 178–180; Jenike MA: "Illness Related to OCD," in *Obsessive-Compulsive Disorders: Theory and Management*, 2nd Edition. Edited by Jenike MA, Baer L, Minichiello WE. Littleton, MA, Year Book Medical, 1991, pp. 39–42.

[6]Jenike MA: "Illness Related to OCD," in *Obsessive-Compulsive Disorders: Theory and Management*, 2nd Edition. Edited by Jenike MA, Baer L, Minichiello WE. Littleton, MA, Year Book Medical, 1991, pp. 39–42.

[7]Hollander E: "Serotonergic Drugs and the Treatment of Disorders Related to Obsessive-Compulsive Disorder," in *Current Treatments of Obsessive-Compulsive Disorder.* Edited by Pato MT, Zohar J. Washington, D.C., American Psychiatric Press, 1991, pp. 178–180.

emission tomography have detected differences in the patterns of regional cerebral glucose metabolism between patients with OCD and patients with trichotillomania.[8]

Comorbidity between trichotillomania and OCD is limited. In a relativily recent study, of 60 adults who chronically pull their hair, 10% had current OCD, and an additional 5% had a history of the disorder.[9] Interestingly, OCD has been reported in 10% of first-degree relatives of patients with trichotillomania.[10] Although OCD may be common among first-degree relatives of patients with OCD,[11] information on familial patterns of impulse-control disorders is not available.

Case Presentation 59
Rituals in Her Mind

Betty, a 15-year-old, was referred for psychiatric evaluation. Betty's condition had been diagnosed as both panic disorder and generalized anxiety disorder, and she was being seen intermittently by a psychiatrist to follow the results of medical therapy prescribed for these disorders. She was also seeing a psychotherapist. Her failure to respond to either of these treatments had led her parents to seek a second opinion.

Most significant in the history was that Betty had received

---

[8] Swedo SE, Rapoport JL, Leonard HL, et al.: "Regional Cerebral Glucose Metabolism of Women With Trichotillomania." *Archives of General Psychiatry* 48:828–833, 1991.

[9] Christenson GA, Mackenzie TB, Mitchell JE: "Characteristics of 60 Adult Chronic Hair Pullers." *American Journal of Psychiatry* 148:365–370, 1991.

[10] Jenike MA: "Illness Related to OCD," in *Obsessive-Compulsive Disorders: Theory and Management*, 2nd Edition. Edited by Jenike MA, Baer L, Minichiello WE. Littleton, MA, Year Book Medical, 1991, pp. 39–42.

[11] Rasmussen SA, Tsuang MT: "Clinical Characteristics and Family History in DSM-III Obsessive-Compulsive Disorder." *American Journal of Psychiatry* 143:317–322, 1986.

extensive, sophisticated, and repeated workups at a major medical center, including testing of her pituitary hormones and for the cause of feelings of weakness and an inability to eat. Anxiety was part of this presenting complex, and she was suspected of having some sort of pituitary problem, causing a variety of somatic complaints. Betty had lost approximately 10 pounds and was described as being quite thin at the beginning of her illness, but there was no associated finding of anorexia nervosa. A sibling 2 years younger than Betty had very severe cerebral palsy, and Betty had to care for her at times. The working hypothesis with regard to Betty's psychological functioning was that her anxiety was a reaction to her sibling's disability and the demands of caring for her. During the last school year Betty had been absent approximately 80% of the time because of her anxiety and the time required for extensive medical testing on both an inpatient and outpatient basis.

At the initial examination Betty appeared to be very slight, anxious, and younger than her stated age of 15 years. She seemed to be of superior intelligence. There was no evidence of psychosis or of a primary depressive disorder. In response to direct questioning, Betty described a very elaborate number system that she had formed in her mind. She noted that she had had ritualized thoughts about numbers for several years but that they had intensified over the past year. In addition, over the past year, Betty had developed a grid system having to do with the location of her house in relation to the location of her school. While sitting in class, she would have to orient herself mentally in relation to where her home was located on this grid.

Betty realized that these thoughts and the "games in her head" were ridiculous but stated that she had been unable to stop herself from performing them during the past year. When asked why she had not told any of her previous examiners about these games, she replied with a laugh, "They didn't ask me." Interviews with Betty's parents revealed that they had been totally unaware of their child's thoughts. Given the very high level of anxiety Betty described and the absence of medical findings, it was apparent that it was this anxiety that had caused her lack of appetite, weight loss, and failure to thrive. There was no evidence of panic disorder or generalized anxiety.

Betty was placed on medication effective in treating OCD, and after only 2 to 3 weeks her anxiety markedly decreased and she was able to return to school. Her anxiety medication was tapered gradually, and she continues to do well on anti-OCD pharmacotherapy.

DSM-IV Diagnosis

Axis I: 300.3   Obsessive-Compulsive Disorder

Discussion

The need to ask direct questions about obsessive and compulsive symptoms has been noted before but is further reinforced by this case. Patients find these symptoms stigmatizing and rarely volunteer the fact that they are occurring unless asked. This is particularly true in children and adolescents. Failure to ask the correct questions in this case resulted in misdiagnosis and prolonged the patient's distress and dysfunction.

This case is also significant for its description of "mental rituals." Mental rituals are compulsions performed strictly in the mind in response to anxiogenic, obsessional thoughts. Like the washing rituals performed by patients obsessed with contamination, mental rituals are anxiolytic. The mental rituals, or "anxiolytic thoughts," in this case were the number games and the patient's efforts to orient herself to the mental map of her location.

Case Presentation 60
The Scent of Obsession

Gwen is a 31-year-old woman referred for follow-up treatment after hospitalization for bipolar disorder with manic symptoms. At the time of her evaluation, her bipolar symptoms are being well controlled by a mood stabilizer and an antidepressant. When asked directly during the interview about obsessions and compulsions, Gwen describes a complex series of intrusive thoughts and rituals that center around perfumes and cosmetics.

When preparing for bed, Gwen is compelled to open and smell every bottle or jar of shampoo, conditioner, and moisturizer on her bathroom shelves. She then proceeds to her bedroom dresser, where she smells every one of her many bottles of perfume and cologne. By the time this task is completed, Gwen begins to fear that she has failed to turn off her gas stove and has to go check all the burners and knobs on the stove. This brings her past the door, where she repeatedly checks the locks. Because she cannot enter either her bathroom or bedroom without performing her smelling rituals again, this ritual proceeds in cycles until hours later she collapses, exhausted. Her fears about leaving the stove turned on are due in part to her conviction that, after her death, people will uncover all her bags and boxes of perfumes and cosmetics.

Often the scent of one particular perfume will "catch" in Gwen's memory, compelling her to go through all her boxes and bags to find all the products made by its manufacturer and clear away those made by other companies. To avoid "contamination," she then wears only products made by that company. Until she gets this "right," Gwen cannot sleep. Frequently, a different scent "catches" in the morning, and then she has to go through the whole routine again, making her late for work.

By the time of the initial interview, Gwen had spent many thousands of dollars acquiring whole lines of cosmetics, shampoos, and other products. She also has a collection of several thousand magazines to help her find them.

Gwen describes episodes during which she became so disgusted that she had to "purge" herself by going through all her perfumes and cosmetics and throwing those she enjoyed most down the drain. Following these episodes, she became frantic and was driven to replace everything she had discarded. On some occasions, Gwen drove to a 24-hour supermarket in a neighboring state where she could buy something that she had to have.

When asked to recall when these behaviors began, she replies, "When I was 9 years old." At the same age, she began pulling out her eyelashes, often while doing "this smelling thing." She still pulls out her eyelashes at times when she feels unusually stressed.

DSM-IV Diagnoses

Axis I: 300.3 Obsessive-Compulsive Disorder

296.46 Bipolar I Disorder, Most Recent Episode Manic, in Full Remission

Discussion

Comorbid OCD and bipolar disorder are somewhat more common than bipolar disorder alone in the population at large; in two series of patients with OCD, the prevalence of bipolar disorder was only 2% to 4%.[12] There exists no consensus on how these disorders may interact. Gordon and Rasmussen described a patient with a 30-year history of OCD whose symptoms lessened during periods of elevated mood but increased when he became depressed.[13] His symptoms showed a distinct seasonality, with euphoria in the fall and winter and depression in the spring and summer. These authors cited other reported cases in which euphoria was associated with improvement in obsessive and compulsive symptoms, and speculated that increased serotonergic neurotransmission during mania may have been responsible. In contrast, Austin et al. found that OCD symptoms in several patients were more severe during manic episodes.[14] In Gwen's case, it is possible to consider the manic episodes during which she would desperately replace her cosmetic supplies to be secondary to OCD.

[12] Rasmussen SA, Tsuang MT: "Clinical Characteristics and Family History in DSM-III Obsessive-Compulsive Disorder." *American Journal of Psychiatry* 143:317–322, 1986; Austin LS, Lydiard RB, Ballenger JC, et al.: "Comorbidity of OCD and Bipolar Affective Disorder." Paper presented at the 144th annual meeting of the American Psychiatric Association, New Orleans, Louisiana, May 1991.

[13] Gordon A, Rasmussen SA: "Mood-Related Obsessive-Compulsive Symptoms in a Patient With Bipolar Affective Disorder." *Journal of Clinical Psychiatry* 49:27–28, 1988.

[14] Austin LS, Lydiard RB, Ballenger JC, et al.: "Comorbidity of OCD and Bipolar Affective Disorder." Paper presented at the 144th annual meeting of the American Psychiatric Association, New Orleans, Louisiana, May 1991.

Another interesting aspect of this case is the strong olfactory component, especially the way in which scents were capable of triggering symptoms, not only of OCD but also of trichotillomania. Although trichotillomania was not included in the diagnosis, it was clearly evident during childhood and is likely still present, at least in remission, at the current time.

CME Test
Chapter 10
Case Presentations 55–60

Please read the six sets of questions (12 questions total) that follow and circle the one best answer for each question on the corresponding answer sheet in the accompanying booklet.

Case Presentation 55: The Boy Who Would Not Behave

55A. Which is *not* a clue that this patient suffers from obsessive-compulsive disorder (OCD)?
  1. His irritable, sullen mood during the psychiatric interview.
  2. His regret that he misses so many classes.
  3. His slowness.

55B. OCD should be considered as a possible cause of behavior problems in a child when
  1. The behavior problems include the yelling of obscenities.
  2. The diagnosis of oppositional defiant disorder has been made.
  3. The behavior problems are associated with seemingly minor interruptions in the child's daily activities.

Case Presentation 56: Obsessed With Her Fears

56A. This patient's avoidance behavior
  1. Should be regarded, in her case, as compulsive or ritualistic behavior.
  2. Was *not* performed to neutralize the anxiety resulting from her obsessive thoughts.
  3. Was triggered by a fear of being attacked by a co-worker at the bank where she worked.

56B. The diagnosis of delusional disorder does not apply to this patient's case partly because
  1. Her persecutory fears were unrelated to her obsessions.
  2. Her fears largely resolved with treatment.
  3. She did not fear anyone or anything specifically.

Case Presentation 57: The Boy Who Collected Soda Cans

57A. This patient's compulsion to collect soda cans
   1. Can be resisted only in the presence of his mother.
   2. Was somewhat masked, as a symptom of OCD, by his pervasive developmental disorder.
   3. Helps him form friendships, because he often interests other children in collecting cans with him.

57B. A clue that this patient has a pervasive developmental disorder is
   1. His inability to keep conversations with his peers going.
   2. His compulsion to pick up soda cans while out walking.
   3. His insistence that any friends he plays with collect soda cans, too.

Case Presentation 58: The Roots of Her Problems

58A. Although trichotillomania is an impulse-control disorder, it is sometimes referred to as an "OCD spectrum disorder" because
   1. It is usually ego-dystonic, unreasonable, and frequently resisted.
   2. Comorbidity of OCD is the rule when trichotillomania is present.
   3. Patterns of regional cerebral glucose metabolism for patients with either disorder are virtually identical.

58B. A probable precipitating factor for this patient's trichotillomania is
   1. The birth of her brother.
   2. Her mother's frequent checking of the roots of her daughter's hair.
   3. Frustration over frequent attempts by others to stop her incessant talking.

Case Presentation 59: Rituals in Her Mind

59A. What key element in this case led to the initial misdiagnosis of anxiety syndrome?
   1. Failure to ask the correct questions.

2. The fact that the patient often took care of her severely disabled sister.
3. The patient's loss of appetite and school absences.

59B. Mental rituals are
1. Mental games that produce pleasurable thoughts once completed.
2. Obsessions associated with guilt feelings.
3. Rituals performed only in the mind, usually in response to anxiogenic, obsessional thoughts.

Case Presentation 60: The Scent of Obsession

60A. Comorbidity of OCD and bipolar disorder
1. Leads to decreased OCD symptoms when the patient is in the manic stage.
2. Is seen with a prevalence of 20% to 30%.
3. Is seen in fewer than 5% of patients with OCD.

60B. In this patient's case, scents were capable of triggering symptoms of
1. OCD and trichotillomania.
2. Euphoria.
3. Bulimia.

Obsessive-compulsive disorder (OCD) is fascinating for those persons who study and treat it, but frustrating and distressing for those sufferers. The *Obsessive-Compulsive Disorder Casebook* has presented many variations on the main theme of OCD, including common and rare comorbidities and obsessive-compulsive spectrum disorders. Although these cases touch on many aspects of OCD, no set of cases is comprehensive. Some important writings on OCD are given in the "Further Reading" listing beginning on p. 181.

Those persons seeking specific information about OCD and the OCD spectrum disorders and about the treatments of these disorders may wish to contact the Obsessive Compulsive Information Center, which is staffed by two master's-level medical librarians and has more than 7,300 OCD citations in a bibliographic program. Paper copies of all cited articles are maintained and will be sent in compliance with copyright laws for a fee to those who request them.

For further information, please contact:

The Obsessive Compulsive Information Center
Dean Foundation for Health, Research and Education
8000 Excelsior Drive, Suite 302
Madison, Wisconsin 53717-1914
Telephone 608-836-8070
FAX 608-836-8033

Information Specialists
Margaret G. Baudhuin, M.L.S.
Bette L. Hartley, M.L.S.

FURTHER READING

Baer L: Behavior therapy for obsessive compulsive disorder in the office-based practice. J Clin Psychiatry 54 (No 6, Suppl):10–15, 1993

Baer L: Getting Control: Overcoming Your Obsessions and Compulsions. Boston, MA, Little, Brown, 1991

Baer L, Jenike MA: Personality disorders in obsessive-compulsive disorder, in Obsessive-Compulsive Disorders: Theory and Management, 2nd Edition. Edited by Jenike MA, Baer L, Minichiello WE. Chicago, IL, Year Book Medical, 1991, pp 76–88

Baxter LR Jr, Schwartz JM, Guze BH, et al: PET imaging in obsessive compulsive disorder with and without depression. J Clin Psychiatry 51 (No 4, Suppl):61–69, 1990

Clomipramine in the treatment of patients with obsessive-compulsive disorder: the Collaborative Study Group. Arch Gen Psychiatry 48:730–738, 1991

Dar R, Greist JH: Behavior therapy for obsessive compulsive disorder. Psychiatr Clin North Am 15:885–894, 1992

De Silva P, Rachman S: Obsessive-Compulsive Disorder: The Facts. New York, Oxford University Press, 1992

Diagnosis and treatment of OCD: a clinician's perspective. J Clin Psychiatry, Vol 54, No 6, Suppl, 1993

Foa EB, Wilson R: Stop Obsessing!: How to Overcome Your Obsessions and Compulsions. New York, Bantam Books, 1991

Goodman WK, McDougle CJ, Barr LC, et al: Biological approaches to treatment-resistant obsessive compulsive disorder. J Clin Psychiatry 54 (No 6, Suppl):16–26, 1993

Goodman WK, Price LH, Rasmussen SA, et al: The Yale-Brown Obsessive Compulsive Scale, I: development, use, and reliability. Arch Gen Psychiatry 46:1006–1011, 1989

Goodman WK, Price LH, Rasmussen SA, et al: The Yale-Brown Obsessive Compulsive Scale, II: validity. Arch Gen Psychiatry 46:1012–1016, 1989

Goodman WK, McDougle CJ, Price LH: Pharmacotherapy of obsessive compulsive disorder. J Clin Psychiatry 53 (No 4, Suppl):29–37, 1992

Greist JH: Treatment of obsessive compulsive disorder: psychotherapies, drugs, and other somatic treatment. J Clin Psychiatry 51 (No 8, Suppl):44–50, 1990

Greist JH: An integrated approach to treatment of obsessive compulsive disorder. J Clin Psychiatry 53 (No 4, Suppl):38–41, 1992

Greist JH: Obsessive Compulsive Disorder: A Guide, Revised Edition. Madison, WI, Obsessive Compulsive Information Center, 1992

Greist JH, Jefferson JW, Marks IM: Anxiety and Its Treatment: Help Is Available. Washington, DC, American Psychiatric Press, 1986

Greist JH, Rapoport JL, Rasmussen SA: Spotting the obsessive-compulsive. Patient Care 24(9):47–50 ff, 1990

Hand I, Goodman WK, Evers U: Obsessive-Compulsive Disorders: New Research Results. New York, Springer-Verlag, 1992

Hollander E (ed): Obsessive-Compulsive Related Disorders. Washington, DC, American Psychiatric Press, 1993

Jenike MA: Illness related to obsessive-compulsive disorder, in Obsessive-Compulsive Disorders: Theory and Management, 2nd Edition. Edited by Jenike MA, Baer L, Minichiello WE. Chicago, IL, Year Book Medical, 1991, pp 39–60

Jenike MA, Rauch SL: Managing the patient with treatment-resistant obsessive compulsive disorder: current strategies. J Clin Psychiatry 55 (No 3, Suppl):11–17, 1994

Jenike MA, Baer L, Minichiello WE (eds): Obsessive-Compulsive Disorders: Theory and Management, 2nd Edition. Chicago, IL, Year Book Medical, 1991

Karno M, Golding JM, Sorenson SB, et al: The epidemiology of obsessive-compulsive disorder in five US communities. Arch Gen Psychiatry 45:1094–1099, 1988

Kim SW, Dysken MW, Katz R: Rating scales for obsessive compulsive disorder. Psychiatric Annals 19:74–79, 1989

March JS, Mulle K, Herbel B: Behavioral psychotherapy for children and adolescents with obsessive-compulsive disorder: an open trial of a new protocol-driven treatment package. J Am Acad Child Adolesc Psychiatry 33:333–341, 1994

Marks IM: Fears, Phobias, and Rituals. New York, Oxford University Press, 1987

Mavissakalian M, Turner SM, Michelson L (eds): Obsessive-Compulsive Disorder: Psychological and Pharmacological Treatment. New York, Plenum, 1985

Montgomery SA: The separate diagnostic status of obsessive-compulsive disorder, in Serotonin-Related Psychiatric Syndromes: Clinical and Therapeutic Links. Edited by Cassano GB, Akiskal HS. London, Royal Society of Medicine Services, 1991, pp 67–72

Murphy DL, Zohar J, Benkelfat C, et al: Obsessive-compulsive disorder as a 5-HT subsystem–related behavioural disorder. Br J Psychiatry 155 (suppl 8):15–24, 1989

Neziroglu F, Yaryura-Tobias JA: Over and Over Again: Understanding Obsessive-Compulsive Disorder. Lexington, MA, Lexington Books, 1991

Obsessive-compulsive spectrum disorders. Psychiatric Annals, Vol 23, No 7, 1993

OCD: comorbidity and management dilemmas. J Clin Psychiatry, Vol 55, No 5, Suppl, 1994

Pato MT, Zohar J (eds): Current Treatments of Obsessive-Compulsive Disorder. Washington, DC, American Psychiatric Press, 1991

Pauls DL: Gilles de la Tourette syndrome and obsessive-compulsive disorder: familial relationships, in Jenike MA, Baer L, Minichiello WE (eds): Obsessive-Compulsive Disorders: Theory and Management, 2nd Edition. Chicago, IL, Year Book Medical, 1991, pp 149–153

Rachman SJ, Hodgson RJ: Obsessions and Compulsions. Englewood Cliffs, NJ, Prentice-Hall, 1980

Rapoport JL: The neurobiology of obsessive-compulsive disorder. JAMA 260:2888–2890, 1988

Rapoport JL (ed): Obsessive-Compulsive Disorder in Children and Adolescents. Washington, DC, American Psychiatric Press, 1989

Rapoport JL: The Boy Who Couldn't Stop Washing: The Experiences & Treatment of Obsessive-Compulsive Disorder. New York, EP Dutton, 1989

Rapoport JL, Leonard HL, Swedo SE, et al: Obsessive compulsive disorder in children and adolescents: issues in management. J Clin Psychiatry 54 (No 6, Suppl):27–29, 1993

Rasmussen SA, Eisen JL: Heterogeneity and coexistence in DSM-III-R obsessive compulsive disorder, in New Directions in Affective Disorders. Edited by Lerer B, Gershon S. New York, Springer-Verlag, 1989, pp 423–427

Rasmussen SA, Eisen JL: Epidemiology and clinical features of obsessive-compulsive disorder, in Jenike MA, Baer L, Minichiello WE (eds): Obsessive-Compulsive Disorders: Theory and Management, 2nd Edition. Chicago, IL, Year Book Medical, 1991, pp 10–27

Rauch SL, Jenike MA: Neurobiological models of obsessive compulsive disorder. Psychosomatics 34:20–32, 1993

Recent advances in bipolar and obsessive compulsive disorders: nature and treatment. J Clin Psychiatry, Vol 51, No 8, Suppl, 1990

Steketee GS: Treatment of Obsessive Compulsive Disorder. New York, Guilford, 1993

Steketee G, White K: When Once Is Not Enough: Help for Obsessive-Compulsives. Oakland, CA, New Harbinger Publications, 1990

Swedo SE, Leonard HL, Rapoport JL: Childhood-onset obsessive compulsive disorder. Psychiatr Clin North Am 15:767–775, 1992

Van-Noppen BL, Pato MT, Rasmussen SA: Learning to Live With Obsessive Compulsive Disorder, 2nd Edition. New Haven, CT, OC Foundation, 1993

Yaryura-Tobias JA, Neziroglu FA: Obsessive-Compulsive Disorders: Pathogenesis, Diagnosis, Treatment. New York, Marcel Dekker, 1983

Zohar J, Insel T, Rasmussen SA (eds): The Psychobiology of Obsessive-Compulsive Disorder. New York, Springer, 1991

CASE PRESENTATION TITLE INDEX

Note. Major diagnostic categories are printed in boldface capital letters (e.g., **EATING DISORDERS**). Subclasses under major diagnostic categories are printed in regular capital letters (e.g., BIPOLAR DISORDERS), and sub-subclasses appear in boldface type (e.g., **Alcohol Use Disorders**). Specific diagnoses are printed in capital and lowercase letters (e.g., Tourette's disorder). Case numbers in boldface type (e.g., **Case 12**) indicate cases in which the sole diagnosis is obsessive-compulsive disorder.

TIC DISORDERS (*see under* **DISORDERS USUALLY FIRST DIAGNOSED IN INFANCY, CHILDHOOD, OR ADOLESCENCE**)

NATIONAL UNIVERSITY LIBRARY   SAN DIEGO